Jenny Whitby is a member of BAWLA (British Amateur Weightlifters Association). She also holds her RSA (exercise), and ITEC (massage) certificates. She is a Health Educator with the LAY section of the Health Education Authority. She has been teaching exercise for over fifteen years and is the energy behind IN HOUSE FITNESS which she set up seven years ago. Her stretch classes were voted the best in London by *Time Out* magazine. Most of her classes are held on a one to one basis. She has trained many exercise teachers who now work for her in and around London. She also holds open and corporate classes. For details, write to her at IN HOUSE FITNESS, 241 Westbourne Grove, London W11 2SE or telephone 071-727-1793.

Jenny has written for *She* magazine, *What Diet*, *Parents*, *Mother Work-Out*, *New Woman* and *Me*. Her first book, *The Prenatal Exercise Handbook* was published in 1989.

GW00586731

COMMENTS FROM CLIENTS

'These exercises give me the energy to help
push my pen further.'
William Shawcross, author

'Jenny's early morning classes give me
the energy I need to carry out my hectic lifestyle
both in business and socially.'
Olga Polizzi, Director, Trusthouse Forte

'Jenny helped me on the road to recovery
after I broke my back in an accident. When the
physiotherapists couldn't do any more, she worked
wonders and gave me back the strength and
flexibility I thought I could never regain!'
John Culman, Senior Vice President,
The Riggs National Bank of Washington

'My morning workouts have given me much more
flexibility and firmness.'
The Hon. Mrs Louise Burness

'I don't know if I love her or hate her,
all I know is that her regimes work for me and without
her I would be the proverbial "slug".'
City Banker (whose sweat has to remain anonymous)

'I can't start my day without her.
I hate her, she kills me but I adore her. She makes me
work and gives me results.'
Azar Nikkhah, antiques dealer

'Without Jenny's exercises I feel like a soggy souflaki.'
Christianna Goulandris, a Mum

'Her workouts are indispensible.'
Sandy Watson-Scott, commericals producer

BELOW THE BELT

Jenny Whitby

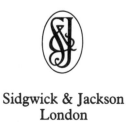

Sidgwick & Jackson
London

First published in Great Britain in 1991
by Sidgwick & Jackson Limited

Copyright © 1991 by Jenny Whitby
Illustrations © 1991 by Neil Greer

ISBN 0-283-99995 0

Cover Design by Splash Studio
Cover Photographs by Ian Potter
Hair by Paco
Make up by Kasha at Enzo Trevi
Shoes by Reebok

Typeset by Florencetype Ltd,
Kewstoke, Avon

Printed and bound in Great Britain by
Mackays of Chatham PLC, Chatham, Kent

for Sidgwick & Jackson Limited
Cavaye Place
London SW10 9PG

CONTENTS

ACKNOWLEDGEMENTS

Thanks to Jo for staying on her programme and letting me have the results I needed, to Edward Abdulnour MD for his help in the section on plastic surgery, to Dr Catherine O'Connor, to Bonnie for taking endless photographs, Neil for his wonderful illustrations, to Marni for hoisting her skirt for my massage illustrations, to all my clients and students and to all those who prefer legs, bum and tums to the 'top bits' and who gave me the incentive to write this book and also to my mum who has a gorgeous pair of legs.

Thank to the following for their tremendous help and guidance with my research:

ASH – Action on Smoking and Health
5–11 Mortimer Street, London W1N 7RH
Tel: 071-637-9843

British Diabetic Association
10 Queen Anne Street, London W1M 0BD
Tel: 071-323-1531
Who published *Countdown* 1989

Nutritionists at Safeway Plc
6 Millington Road, Hayes, Middlesex UB3 4AY
Tel: 081-848-8744

The Times

The Sunday Times

Surgeon Lieutenant Jarmulowicz and Surgeon Commander Buchanan,
Department of Pathology at the Royal Naval Hospital in Haslar
'Exertional Hyperpyrexia: Case report and review of pathophysiological mechanisms'

District Dietitians at St Thomas' Hospital
London SE1 7EH

William S. Beckett, MD et al
'Heat Stress Associated with the use of Vapor-Barrier Garments'
– *Journal of Occupational Medicine*/Volume 28, No 6, June 1986

Sports Documentation Centre at The University of Birmingham

Health & Fitness Magazine
40 Bowling Green Lane, London EC1R 0NE

Auriel Mott at *The Vitamin Connection* January/February 1990 issue

The staff at Nigel Benn's office

Health Education Authority Look After Yourself Project Centre,
Christ Church College, Canterbury, Kent CT1 1QU
Tel: 0227-455564

Sport & Recreational Studies Department at Staffordshire Polytechnic

Harry Shapiro at The Institute for the study of Drug Dependence
1 Hatton Place, London EC1N 8ND
Tel: 071-430-1991

Mr Menzies Campbell, the Liberal Democrats' spokesman on sport

McCance & Widdowson's *The Composition of Foods* by A.A. Paul and
D.A.T. Southgate

BAWLA (British Amateur Weightlifters Association)
3 Iffley Turn, Oxford

British Medical Journal, Volume 295, 24th October 1987

General Council and Register of Osteopaths
56 London Street, Reading, Berkshire
Tel: 0734-576585

British School of Osteopaths
1–4 Suffolk Street, London SW1 Y1HG
Tel: 071-930-9254

British Association of Aesthetic Plastic Surgeons,
Royal College of Surgeons, 35–43 Lincolns Inn Fields, London
Tel: 071-405-2234

FOREWORD

A few years ago, depressed and horrified at the amount of cellulite on my 'below the belt' areas, I embarked on a dedicated anti-cellulite regime. I was delighted – and also surprised – that the cellulite eventually disappeared, but not so happy to note that where I once had lumps and bumps, I now had flab.

What to do? I had previously tried aerobics and yoga, with no noticeable success. I am highly allergic to all forms of exercise, yet I was vain enough to want to be firm and taut.

The answer to my dilemma was Jenny Whitby. She became my personal exerciser and together we worked on the recalcitrant areas. Her programme was tough and at times painful – but it succeeded brilliantly. After six weeks of doing her anti-flab exercises daily, the difference was astonishing. For the first time in two decades, I had wonderful (for me) wobble-free thighs and bum.

And for somebody who normally finds it almost impossible to find the motivation to work out regularly, this *was* an achievement. But it was all thanks to Jenny.

Not everybody can book up Jenny personally, of course, but this book is the next best thing. It conveys her bubbly personality and positive attitude – essential attributes for the successful exercise teacher – and also her sound anatomical knowledge, also vital for a self-help exercise programme.

The dietary and anti-cellulite advice given is also spot-on.

Her programme proves that you are never too old, never too flabby, never too sedentary, to regain muscle tone and the figure of your youth. None of the exercises here are beyond the range of the ordinarily able-bodied person – and it's wonderful to see visible results achieved so quickly.

Liz Hodgkinson

1
INTRODUCTION

When was the last time you had a compliment on the firmness of your bottom, the flatness of your stomach and the shapeliness of your legs? Yesterday? Last week? A few years ago? When you were at school? Or can't you remember? If you come into the last three categories, read on: you need to!

This book is aimed at tackling the 'biggest' problem areas of females and some of the prominent yet saggy bits on males. We women are lucky in that we can disguise our basic shape tremendously with clothes which make us feel fantastic and we can spend a fortune on beautiful underwear. Men are less fortunate in hiding their floppy bits: they usually hang over the top of their trouser waistband! But if, underneath all these stunning garments, our flesh is loose and flabby – what a letdown. Stunning underwear will look terrible on a body full of cellulite and loose flab. Cheap underwear can look – and feel – superb on a firm body. It's not the top layer that counts, it's the bits underneath!

I have one client in the middle of a fairly hot romantic involvement; the only thing which is keeping her lycra on is her worry that her body is flabby and she daren't let her boyfriend see her without any clothes on. She is determined and he is eager! Needless to say, she works hard at both her diet and her daily exercise, and they are proving successful – I hope the relationship lasts long enough for the results to come to light! Another client of mine flatly refused to go on a sailing holiday with her husband and friends because she was too embarrassed to bare her legs. It almost wrecked her marriage. She worked on my programme; now she's toned up, and they're all happy!

OVERCOMING YOUR GENES
We inherit our physical make-up, in one form or another, via our genes. Take, for instance, bunions and varicose veins: if one of your parents has these, you are more likely to inherit them than if neither has. Some of us inherit features directly from one or both parents; some of us skip a generation and go one step further back to inherit a grandparent's features (rarely the best). Mother Nature can sometimes be cruel but it's up to us to trick her, to make the most of our best features and try to knock the worst ones on the head.

Some people inherit genes that produce large amounts of fat and cellulite on the thighs, bottom and stomach. Your mother's legs may be perfect; if you can remember your grandmother's, they may have been full of fatty cellulite. Your sisters may have inherited your mother's shapely legs while you may be unlucky enough to have inherited your grandmother's, in which case you have a great deal of work on your hands (or, more appropriately, your legs!). Look on the bright side, though: you could have inherited your father's, in which case you could be in real trouble, especially if you happen to be female! However, there's no point in dwelling on the past. If you've got floppy bits and it doesn't worry you, fine – some partners find it a turn-on; if you've got them and they upset you and your partner doesn't find it particularly inviting, *and* you are willing to work extremely hard to get them toned up, this book is for you.

This is not an easy programme by any means and it does take time. Forget all those promises of results in hours – if you want lasting results it takes much longer; but you should notice a marked difference in about three weeks and a definite improvement in firmness in six.

WHAT IS CELLULITE?

Cellulite is a fatty deposit beneath the skin, most common on the hips and thighs, though it can occur elsewhere. Run your fingers down your thighs or bottom: if you see an uneven, dimpled effect under the skin – you've got cellulite! Approximately eight out of ten women suffer from the problem, which is related to hormone levels and the body's mechanisms for breaking up fats. Around the time of a period, your oestrogen level is lower than usual, which may make you feel rather bloated: pinch your flesh now and you will probably see a few dimples, rather like the magnified skin of an orange. Again – cellulite. If you are or have been taking the contraceptive pill, my findings suggest that cellulite will settle upon you at some time.

Men, too, suffer from cellulite, despite what some 'experts' have said in the past, though it is often less apparent as men's skin is slightly thicker than women's, which to an extent hides the problem. It does seem to be true, though, that far fewer of them are blessed with it. On men cellulite usually settles on their middles (the beer bellies), around the waist (if it can be found) and on the inner thighs. I notice it more on men whose weight alters drastically. I have one male client who can put on 5 lb over a weekend (and lose it in a couple of days by virtually starving – *not* a good method, as I shall explain in chapter 2): needless to say, he turns into something resembling a lump of dough. It's only when I read the riot act, throw a tantrum, give a lecture on heart-related disease and threaten never to return that he pulls himself up and gets back into a routine. My male clients never cease to amaze me: they are like children.

But apart from playing with toys, they play with their health: this is like playing Russian Roulette and I like them all too much to let them disintegrate prematurely into a pile of dust. I find screaming at them most effective. I don't recommend you do it, though: after all, I can leave after an hour, you may be stuck with yours 24 hours a day!

Why are women troubled with cellulite so much more than men? It seems our hormones have a lot to answer for – we carry more fat than men as food reserves and protection, mainly round our reproductive organs. On some of us, this 'protection' has rather gone overboard and swamped us! During pregnancy, most women notice the distribution of fat getting worse, with fatty layers increasing especially round the waist, bottom and thighs. If, after the birth of the child, the body is not exercised and is left to 'wallow', those fatty layers will remain. Only a great deal of hard work will shift the excess fat. However, no strong abdominal work should be attempted until at least six weeks after the birth and only then when the post-natal check up has been carried out by your doctor.

Before embarking on any exercise programme after the birth of a child, I would encourage any new Mum to have a check up with an osteopath, as the back alignment may have altered slightly. To find a good osteopath, look for the leters DO, MRO, after the name: these signify the proper professional qualifications. There are some osteopaths who have 'qualified' after 'crash' or correspondence courses; I find this difficult to comprehend and personally I wouldn't touch them with a bargepole. Your body is too precious to be manipulated by someone who doesn't really know what they are doing. Therefore, you must ensure the person of your choice knows his or her work thoroughly. If in doubt, contact the General Council and Register of Osteopaths, 56 London Street, Reading, Berkshire (tel. 0734 576585) or the British School of Osteopathy, 1–4 Suffolk Street, London SW1Y 1HG (tel. 071 930 9254).

EXCESS AND WHAT TO DO ABOUT IT

Generally speaking, the ideal proportion of fat on a woman is 20–28 per cent of body weight – 15–22 per cent for a man. Usually the percentage is much higher, and if that excess fat is carried in the form of cellulite, it will look ugly and ageing and feel uncomfortable, the spare flesh moving as you walk and continuing to move once you've stopped!

So how do we reduce this percentage? The answer is simple: a good, well-balanced diet, massage, lots of exercise which keeps you moving, and keeping depression at bay. Easier said than done? Absolutely! However, if you are serious about ridding yourself of a major problem you will work at it, especially when you start to see results, and the folds become firm flesh!

You must realize that the older you are the harder it is to get back into shape; however, it is never impossible. Once you have recognised the problem and decided to exercise, if you want lasting results you have to work at the programme on a regular basis.

It is no good relying on a few muscle contractions alone to tone up your anatomy: you are gong to have to watch your diet too. In tackling cellulite, foods to avoid include dairy produce, stodgy puddings, cakes, fatty meats, sugar and added salt, and you should watch your drinks too: problems here are coffee, tea, alcohol and too much undiluted fruit juice. Many of the people I have seen with a cellulite problem – both men and women – have been overweight as a result of too many business lunches washed down with wine or beer and topped up by another meal in the evening. (One glass of wine or beer a day is just about OK; but if you can cut even this out, so much the better!) If the body takes in masses of fatty foods, it will obviously store these in the form of fat. If the body takes in masses of sugary foods, these too end up as fat if not used. Imagine, if you will, eating a 45 g chocolate bar. Of the total, 13.6 g is pure fat; 29.9 g is carbohydrate; the tiny remainder is protein. On the wrapper it will probably say that the bar will supply energy – of course it will: instant energy! Certainly energy comes from fat and carbohydrates, and we need it as 'fuel' and to preserve the elasticity of the skin. But we only use as much as we need: the rest goes into store, which means that if you don't burn it off by exercising, it will end up on your waist, bottom, thighs . . .

If you visit your doctor with a cellulite problem, he or she will probably dismiss it. The doctor doesn't see you as being ill – which you're not – and therefore can't administer a cure. You will probably be told to go away and make the most of your better qualities. So off you go, feeling very low and dejected. I have had clients who have turned to me in sheer desperation. They have become incredibly distressed because of their physical appearance, with legs or tums or bums (or all three) smothered in 'orange-peel' textured skin. For them to be told there is no cure is extremely distressing. They (both men and women) see youth as a threat and tend to lose their self-confidence. They feel ugly and 'over the hill'. They feel as if the ageing process has descended on them prematurely. To tell these people that there is nothing wrong and to go away as there is no 'cure' is adding to their mental distress.

I make no promises that my programme will rid your body of cellulite totally and forever, but I do urge you to try it. My students have had fantastic results. You can only benefit. As I've mentioned before, though, it's no easy option: you will only reap the benefits by sweating and working; and by following a sensible diet which includes plenty of raw fresh fruit and vegetables. But what have you got to lose?

CELLULITE AND CIRCULATION

There is a circulatory condition called Reynauld's Disease, a hereditary complaint more prevalent in women than in men, and a problem I suffer from. The extremities – fingers and toes – turn purple then white and freeze in cold conditions. It seems the blood supply just doesn't want to reach these areas. It can be painful, and winter months become agonizing as we battle against the elements trying to keep the extremities warm.

A large percentage of my clients with cellulite were women and a large group of them had serious circulatory problems. Apart from bad circulation in the fingers and toes, their bottoms seemed to be forever cold. Bottoms tend to be one of the main problem areas for cellulite, so it seems there could well be a connection between Reynauld's Disease and cellulite. If my hypothesis is correct, it makes good sense to boost the circulation as much as possible to burn off the fatty pockets and to tone up the muscles beneath. So while cellulite may be a hereditary problem, it need not be one you are stuck with. If you exercise properly, and are prepared to work hard at it, you should notice good results. You have more to gain than to lose (apart from fat!). But if you do nothing to shift them, cellulite and fat could be with you forever.

THE IMPORTANCE OF EXERCISE

To shift your cellulite you need to do the *right kind* of exercise. Yoga may well improve your flexibility but it won't get rid of fatty cellulite pockets, nor will it tone up the muscles enough. An hour of solid aerobics will make you sweat buckets but that won't get rid of the cellulite either. What is needed is a good combination of a certain amount of aerobic exercise where the pulse will be raised and a good balance of stretching and strengthening exercises to work the muscles and to help burn off the fatty layer.

Don't expect immediate results: you will probably not notice any real change for at least three weeks, even with regular work – but imagine the difference in six or more!

It seems cellulite will settle in the unsightly fatty pockets when the circulation becomes sluggish. If the circulation can be improved, the cellulite will be reduced. So how long do you need to exercise for to get rid of it? This basically depends again on your inherited genes. If you grew up with cellulite, you will never really get rid of it and I don't make rash promises that you will make it disappear as if by magic overnight by following this regime. However, I *can* promise that you can get it down to a minimum if you keep to your sensible diet and work extremely hard on your exercise programme.

Exercise cannot be taken lightly. When I was running – in training for marathons – cycling, swimming *and* taking an exercise class every day, I was at the peak of my physical fitness with a bum and tum of steel. When the marathon training finished and I decided to take it easy for a while, the muscle tone slackened and floppy bits started to appear. Not too much, because being aware of what could happen, I still exercised in one way or another; but I was not doing enough to retain the physical firmness I wanted.

I didn't gain weight with the decrease in exercise; but while the weight didn't increase, the floppy bits did, especially on my thighs and bum which tend to be problem areas on most of us. It seemed I either had to run marathons (the training for which I now found exhausting especially as I was teaching much more) or do something else to bash the creeping flab. And the problem became noticeably worse as I got older. You hit the big four-O and suddenly bits seem to indent where you want them to bulge and bulge where you want them to go in. So I had to devise a regime quickly, and one that wasn't going to pummel me into the ground. To give me more incentive, my boyfriend is a leg and bum man and I'm vain enough to care about what I look like starkers. I had to keep all my bits firm. I didn't want to be the only geriatric in the 'Top Shop' and 'Way In' changing rooms with creases (everybody looks at your shape in open-plan changing rooms!) and I had no desire to carry around extra 'flab' and to feel I couldn't wear shorts or short skirts because of lumps of loose flesh. I really do feel that no matter how old you are, it's never too late to get into shape, and you can never be too vain to want what slightly younger people have – firm bits!

I decided if I wasn't careful and didn't work hard enough quickly enough, I could see myself turning into a barrel of lard. Even though I was teaching many classes – as many as six a day – I wasn't working on myself. While I was teaching others on a one-to-one basis how to reach their physical peak, I was in fact leaving me out. I tended to concentrate so much on watching what they were doing and seeing they exercised correctly that I had little time left for myself. Even though I'd do a couple of leg lifts or bum firmers here and there, it wasn't consistent. This goes to show there are no easy ways out, even when you know the ropes! It's so easy to take short cuts – work on clients, show them what to do, then have a rest while they work up a sweat. They got the results I wanted them to have, but I was easing down on myself and I found that exercising bits here and there had absolutely no effect; you have to work at your 45 minutes in one fell swoop.

With the regime I'll show you in this book you really can battle with the ageing process and keep highlighting your hair all the way to the pension book without feeling like mutton dressed as lamb. So prepare yourself, and go for it. If you want something badly enough, you'll work: and I warn you, it is an uphill struggle! (Talking of which, hill walking is brilliant for the thighs and bottom . . .) But it's worth it! There is no point in attempting a programme half-heartedly. You have to be determined to work and work hard on a regular basis. My clients pay a fortune for personal tuition. If you have the motivation, you can obtain the same results for the price of this book!

GETTING RESULTS

Results take time. Don't go by how much weight you lose; go by the centimetres you lose. For long-lasting results, you should exercise *and* diet to prevent your body from sagging. A client told me a story about a woman at a dinner party who had lost a tremendous amount of weight and was proud that she had managed it without any exercise – she 'didn't need it', it was 'a waste of time'. However, as she reached across the table, she actually had to hold the underside of her upper arm to prevent the hanging flesh dangling in her second course. This shows you how important it is to exercise when dieting. If you don't, you'll have sagging bits all over the place and they might not be limited to dangling over the supper table!

Thanks to my 'guinea pigs' (which I will tell you about in the next chapter), I was able to prove my point that just 45 minutes a day will transform you. The first in line was my niece Joanne, whom I almost bullied on to the programme. She was 16 years old, 5'6", and weighed 14½ stone: a very big girl! However, being a kindly aunt, I took her under my wing, bribed her and gradually eased into the programme. It cost me the price of two tickets to see Prince!

Twelve weeks later she'd lost 30 lb and shrunk from a size 18 to a size 12. She looks fantastic. At one time she had little interest in clothes, usually hiding herself away in voluminous black folds of material. She wouldn't wear trousers at all. Now she goes on shopping sprees and helps spend her father's money on brighter, younger styles. Needless to say, while her ego goes up, his bank balance goes down!

Obviously Jo did go through bouts of depression. Some weeks there seemed to be a barrier of boredom and lethargy when she wanted to turn to the crisp bag for comfort. This she was allowed to do as long as she only took out one or two and savoured them; but no more, otherwise I'd wash my hands of her. She was terrific. She religiously locked herself away in her bedroom to do her exercises daily. She always knew that I was only a telephone call away, if ever she needed to talk. Not surprisingly, both our telephone bills rocketed during that period. However, it was well worth it when we saw the results!

Before starting on her programme, Jo would feel exhausted at having to do anything more energetic than getting in and out of bed. Now she was beginning to feel energized and wanted to 'boogie': life had suddenly become more interesting. The programme was working.

Again, I must stress that it is more important to measure than weigh yourself. Scales can be depressing and if you see little or no weight loss, you are more tempted to go on a binge – a vicious, self-destructive circle. So weigh yourself at the beginning of your proposed programme then again at the end; in the interim hide the scales away or give them to the Oxfam shop!

2
YOUR DIET

THE GUINEA PIGS

For this programme, I selected a group of 'guinea pigs' from various of my clients – both private clients I was seeing on a one-to-one basis and students who came en masse from the exercise classes. They were all intelligent men and women from a variety of jobs – secretaries, bankers, lawyers, writers, lab technicians, film producers, physiotherapists, etc. I put the students into three groups – those who exercised once a week for one hour, those who exercised for half an hour every other day, and those who exercised for 45 minutes every day. Then I asked each of them to complete a questionnaire giving details of their diet, lifestyle, work and leisure activities.

These people were desperate to tone up. Beneath the slinky tights on the women and the shorts that came below the stomach bulge on the men could be seen the outline of wrinkly pockets of cellulite and floppy, loose flesh. This intelligent bunch presumed that just by cutting down a bit on their food intake – taking a smaller piece of cake instead of the biggest – and exercising now and again, metamorphosis would take place. However, it's not as easy as that. To tone up and rid the body of toxins demands a combination of the correct exercise, regular massage and a good balanced diet which doesn't leave you feeling hungry, depressed, lethargic and guilty.

The women with a cellulite problem were all shapes and sizes and had all taken the contraceptive pill, for periods ranging from five to twenty years. The older they were, the worse the problem was becoming. Those who exercised once a week noticed no difference in firmness; those who exercised for half an hour every other day saw minimal changes; but those who exercised for 45 minutes every day noticed huge improvements in the fatty pockets and a definite increase in firmness, especially from the waist to the knees. The men with a cellulite problem were the ones who binged and then lost weight drastically. They usually did no exercise; if they did, it would be in sudden bursts, when they'd become very competitive.

THE QUESTIONNAIRES

The questionnaire I handed out asked each client to write down everything that passed his or her lips in one typical day, and at the same time to record mood swings. I wanted honest answers and told them to eat normally. Everything had to be logged.

When the completed questionnaires came back I was amazed at what I read. Despite the amount of media exposure given to dietary dos and don'ts, these people, who ranged from averagely to extremely intelligent, had little or no idea of where they were going wrong in their eating habits. There were endless cups of tea and coffee, crispbreads, apples and cheese but hardly any fresh raw vegetables or other fruit.

This made me want to find out what was being eaten during a typical week, so I distributed another round of questionnaires. This time I also asked for information such as height, weight and various measurements; also whether the women had ever taken the contraceptive pill and if so for how long. I was intrigued as to what was happening to these students, both in diet and in exercise. Quite of few of them only attended an exercise class once a week and although they assured me they worked out at home by themselves, I couldn't figure out why they weren't getting better results.

Once again the completed questionnaires were returned with mood swings noted alongside what had been eaten. Below are a few examples, each with a short comment from me at the end. I have chosen the sheets at random and in each case have taken just one day from seven – the food intake for the week followed a similar pattern to the one I have chosen. You might find quite a few of them familiar.

E.D. Tries to eat sensibly and is cutting down her food intake; feels overweight and has a cellulite problem. Realizes she drinks more coffee than she should, but her office has a free coffee machine! Desk-bound job; works out once a week when she has time.

Time	Intake	Mood
8.00	Cornflakes with milk and sugar, cup of tea	hungry
10.30	Coffee (with sweetener)	habit
11.30	Coffee (with sweetener)	thirsty
12.00	Chilli with rice, coffee (with sweetener)	hungry
4.30	Coffee (with sweetener)	habit
6.00	Coffee (with sweetener) Mars bar	tired
8.00	Ham and cheese sandwich, coffee (with sweetener)	tired
10.00	Tea (with sweetener)	thirsty

(No fresh fruit nor vegetables; too much caffeine.)

J.N. Trying to lose weight, gets bored, works out once a week usually. Cellulite problem on legs and bottom.

Time	Intake	Mood
8.00	Slice of toast and butter, orange juice	hungry
9.30	Coffee (white with sweetener)	habit
11.00	Coffee (white with sweetener)	
noon	Diet Coke	hungry
1.30	3 crispbreads, cheese spread, banana, Bounty bar	hungry
3.30	Diet Coke	thirsty
6.00	Small tin spaghetti bolognaise, slice bread, Diet Coke, coffee (white with sweetener)	hungry and rushing
7.00	Sugar icing (quite a bit)	Icing a cake
10.30	Cold meat sandwich	Hadn't been eating properly and needed something solid

(No fresh vegetables, diet heavy and boring.)

A.K. Watching her weight, becomes easily depressed. Has a sedentary office job, works out once a week. Excess weight on the tummy, legs and bottom with a cellulite problem.

Time	Intake	Mood
7.30	½ pint water	OK
8.30	1 bagel with medium fat curd cheese and jam, juice of 3 oranges, 1 pt water	
11.00		tearful
12.30	Chicken curry, rice and veg., 1 piece of apple cake, can sparkling apple juice	hungry
3.00	Handful Japanese rice crackers	indifferent
3.30	Hot chocolate	unhappy
4.00	½ pt mineral water	
6.30	Packet of crisps, 1½ pts mineral water	bored
9.30	Pasta carbonara (bacon, egg yolks, cream), 2 glasses red wine	tired

(Lots of carbohydrates and fat. Nothing raw, although the fresh orange juice is on the right track; could increase fresh fruit and vegetables and cut out the snacks. Water intake good.)

A.F. Wants to be fitter and lose a few pounds. Has bad circulation. Loose flab problem on bottom and thighs.

Time	Intake	Mood
7.00	150 g hazelnut yoghurt, glass orange juice	tired
7.30	Cup of coffee (white with sweetener)	alert
10.00	Water	OK
11.30	Coffee (white with sweetener)	preoccupied
12.30	Coffee (white with sweetener)	relaxed
3.00	Coffee (white with sweetener)	cold
4.00	Coffee (white with sweetener)	preoccupied
5.00	Coffee (white with sweetener)	bored
8.00	Tuna, broadbeans, baked potato with butter, apple, white coffee, Mars bar	hungry
11.30	Coffee (white with sweetener)	tired

(Boring diet, again no raw vegetables. Goes too long without eating. Retains sweetness level; too much caffeine.)

J.N. Wants to lose a few pounds but gets bored with diets. Heavy on the bottom, legs and tummy. Lots of cellulite.

Time	Intake	Mood
9.00	Grapefruit	hungry
10.00	Four biscuits, cup of tea	hungry
1.30	Diet Coke	thirsty
4.30	Slice of bread and butter	
7.00	Take-away: spring roll, rice, sweet and sour pork, prawns with egg, chicken, beef noodles, glass of wine	bloated
9.00	Slice of cake	relaxed
10.00	Another slice of cake, orange squash	relaxed

(What a diet: high in fat and hardly the right material to help her lose weight! Nothing fresh or raw, too much stodge, not enough liquids.)

E.N. Heavy on the bottom and legs with cellulite problem. Sits at a desk for most of her working day.

Time	Intake	Mood
10.00	Orange juice	thirsty

noon	Orange squash	thirsty
1.00	3 slimline bitter lemon drinks, glass of wine, few handfuls of peanuts	thirsty
4.00	Roast pork, waldorf salad, potato salad, coleslaw, cottage cheese, brown roll and butter, fresh fruit salad and cream, glass of lemonade	hungry
4.30	Glass of lemonade, packet of peanuts	thirsty
7.00	Cup of tea	thirsty
8.00	Few more peanuts . . .	relaxed
9.00	2 boiled eggs and soldiers	hungry
10.30	Several chocolates	bored

(Another boring diet, high in fats, though she did choose fresh fruit salad. Should try substituting mineral water for lemonade. Could also try to cut down on salty snacks.)

R.L. He has a sedentary job and tries to exercise three times a week. Heavy round the middle with a cellulite problem on the tummy and inner thighs.

Time	*Intake*	*Mood*
9.00	Cup of tea	quiet
9.30	Cup of tea	livens up
10.30	2 rolls (cheese and tuna) cup of tea	OK
12.00	Cup of tea	low
2.00	1 tuna roll	livens up
2.30	Cup of tea	
3.30	Cup of tea	
5.00	Cup of tea	
5.30		tired
7.00	Cup of tea	relaxed
7.30	Fish and chips, cup of tea	livens up
10.00	Can of beer	
12.00	Cup of tea	tired

(Typical boring, rushed diet; tea, tea and more tea with stodge and chips thrown in as a 'filler' – hardly the diet to promote energy.)

A.F. Desk-bound job. Lots of looseness but minimal cellulite.

Time	*Intake*	*Mood*
7.30	Slice wholemeal toast and butter, orange juice, mug of coffee	
10.30	White coffee	frustrated; excuse to leave the desk

21

Time	Intake	Mood
12.30	White coffee	bored
1.30	Cup of hot chocolate	happy
3.30	White coffee	bored
7.30	Baked potato with butter and savoury mince, coffee	hungry
10.30	White coffee	tired
		bored

(Boredom seems to be the order of the day here, with endless cups of coffee which don't seem to be serving any purpose other than an excuse to get away from the desk. Goes too long without eating; has lost interest in and enthusiasm for herself.)

J.N. Heavy from the waist down with cellulite on tum, bum and thighs.

Time	Intake	Mood
9.00	Orange juice	hungry
10.30	Coffee with sweetener	habit
11.30	Diet Coke	thirsty
12.30	Diet Coke	thirsty
1.30	Chicken salad, yogurt	hungry
3.00	Coffee with sweetener	thirsty
4.00	Diet Coke	bored
6.30	Chunk of cheese	starving
7.00	Chicken supreme, broad beans, peas, carrots, green beans. Yogurt. Diet Coke	
8.30	Apple and cheese, coffee with sweetener	bored
9.30	8 chocolates	bored

(Starts off with good intentions but see how she turns to the apple and cheese and then to the binge on chocolates. Lots of diet drinks which retain the 'sweet tooth' and caffeine which stimulates the appetite.)

F.G. Small-framed but heavy from the waist down with lots of looseness.

Time	Intake	Mood
9.00	Slice of toast with butter, orange juice	hungry
10.30	Coffee with sweetener	habit
11.30	Diet Coke	thirsty
12.30	Coffee with sweetener	hungry
1.30	3 crispbreads, low fat cheese spread, 2 tomatoes, yogurt; Diet Coke	hungry, thirsty
7.30	Apple	hungry

8.00	Diet lasagne, peas, carrots, green beans, Diet Coke, Kit Kat	hungry, thirsty
10.30	Orange squash	thirsty

(Spends most of the day feeling hungry and thirsty but doesn't ever turn to water, always the diet drinks and coffee, which, as you can see, scream at the taste buds to hold on to sweetness.)

A.B. Hectic lifestyle, finds it hard to relax. He rushes round a lot – meetings, business lunches etc. – and sleeps very little (three or four hours a night). Cat-naps whenever possible! Cellulite on the stomach and inner thighs.

Time	*Intake*	*Mood*
6.30	Freshly squeezed grapefruit juice, black coffee	tired
8.00	Coffee	tired
9.30	Coffee	OK
11.00	Coffee	OK
12.30	Steak, green beans, potatoes, fruit salad, ¾ bottle of wine, black coffee	full
3.00	Coffee	lethargic
4.30	Coffee	frantic
5.00	Packet of nuts, coffee	OK
6.00	Glass of wine	OK
7.30	Parma ham, melon, lamb chops, salad, potatoes, carrots, crème brulée, 3 glasses wine, coffee	full
9.00	Brandy, coffee	
11.00	Coffee	tired
12.00	Diet Coke	tired
1.00	Fruit juice	restless

(Far too much coffee, too heavy a diet, too much alcohol.)

All these diets go wrong in that they are basically boring and loaded with carbohydrates teamed with fats. Also, the respondents tended to have drastic mood swings through frustration, boredom, lethargy, tearfulness and the last one was positively neurotic!

Carbohydrates are relatively low in calories, as is protein – both at 4 calories per gram. Fats on the other hand, are high at 9 calories per gram. It is when carbohydrates are teamed with fats that the number of calories goes sky-high. Take, for example, a baked potato with butter and savoury mince. The baked potato is good; it's the fat in the butter and again in the savoury mince which will add the excess calories. If your food intake is more than your body needs and you tend not to move very

23

much, i.e. not to use up much energy, the surplus will be stored as fat. If you don't burn up the excess fats and carbohyrates, you will become more rotund and 'soft' and will feel more sluggish. The less your body does in the form of exercise, the less it will want to do and the slower your metabolic rate will become. As most of my guinea pigs had desk-bound jobs, they couldn't get rid of the added fat by working it off.

Bad diets also seem to lead to boredom, both at work and socially. As you can see, the majority of those on the trial readily turned to the coffee machine, diet drinks or a 'treat' in the form of a chocolate bar or cake. They tended to choose 'comfort' food which is usually lacking in vitamins and minerals. If you choose a piece of fruit instead of cake or a chocolate bar, you will experience slow-release energy instead of feeling lethargic and storing yet another 'pleat'. You will also feel fuller. Of course it's easier said than done, but give it a try! Fruit will satisfy your appetite for a while because you're eating 'bulk' and taking in fibre. One whole orange is equal to the juice of three oranges. As soon as the fruit is juiced the fibre content plummets. So if you turn to fruit juice you may quench your thirst for a little while but you'll still have the hunger pangs. As you can see from the sample diet sheets, my guinea pigs were eating hardly any fresh fruit or raw vegetables, usually because of rushed itineraries. This has an important bearing on the fat problem, because fresh fruit and vegetables have a lot of filling power for relatively few calories – as well as many essential nutrients missing from most snack and convenience foods.

On the whole these people drank very little water, preferring lots of tea, coffee and diet drinks. These would give an instant boost to the energy level, but the effect would be short-lived, so they would then turn to another drink or another treat to get the 'hype' they needed to carry on. This drinking pattern has two disadvantages. First, we *need* water! Water is an essential part of our bodies, making up half of our body weight. It also helps our bodies cool down when we sweat, acting as an inbuilt thermostat. We can survive for weeks without food but only up to four days without water! Admittedly, we do get a certain amount of water from different drinks but those such as coffee act as a diuretic, actually taking from the body water which it so desperately needs. You will probably notice this after drinking a cup or two when you have to visit the loo more often! You may also feel quite hyped up and can in fact become caffeine-sensitive – extremely 'edgy'.

Secondly, when you keep taking sweetened drinks your taste buds become used to the same level of sweetness and crave more, whether in the form of sugars or artificial sweeteners. OK, the calories are usually zero in diet drinks but you still have the disadvantage of remaining hooked on the same sweetness level. Also, more often than not, the low-sugar versions of these drinks still have the same caffeine content as the originals, so go on tempting you to turn to chocolate bars etc.: caffeine is a stimulant and will activate your appetite, making you want to eat more.

Remember, when you take an excess of sugar in the diet, it turns to fat and *fat stores as fat!*

I was horrified at much of what I learnt from these questionnaires. The ones who desperately wanted to lose weight and rid their bodies of 'excess baggage' were the ones who were eating worst and bingeing, usually on the wrong type of food: quickie snacks, crisps, peanuts and chocolates – the sort that are supposed to help you 'work, rest and play'; they wanted to rest all right, they had no energy: just surplus stores of fat! Those who exercised once a week tended to have the worst diets and lifestyles; it almost seemed that they were doing their weekly exercise as a penance for a particular way of life.

Diets, it seemed, definitely needed taking in hand. All my guinea pigs were intelligent but their basic knowledge of nutrition didn't rate highly on the one to ten scale! They knew that coffee would keep them awake and chocolate would make them happy. They seemed to be surviving on black coffee – on average five cups a day with artificial sweeteners – apples, cheese, grapefruit (which they seemed to think had powers to burn off the fat: it doesn't!), slimming biscuits and the odd binge of chocolate and booze. All this wasn't helping them: in fact, quite the opposite. For example, most of the cheeses they chose to eat were of the hard variety which are also in the high-salt category: Cheddar, Parmesan, Stilton, etc. Salt retains fluid and the saltier the food, the more thirsty you become. You may have noticed the type of snacks which pubs offer. They are mainly salty – crisps, peanuts etc. – to make you drink more. The more you drink with a salty product, the more fluid your body will retain and the harder your kidneys have to work to filter out the toxins. This is why you have to pee much more when you drink alcohol, because the kidneys are working much harder than if you are drinking pure water.

REFORMING YOUR EATING HABITS

Our eating patterns are set down in childhood. If we are offered sweets and ice creams as rewards for being good – or to bribe us into being good – we take this association with us as we grow older. How many times have you felt depressed and to cheer yourself up turned to 'comfort' food in the form of a cream cake, chocolate bar, ice cream, etc? The last thing we want as a treat is a stick of celery! The treats are endless. So are the calories.

If you have children, give them fruit or nuts or raw vegetables when they want a treat, and make them aware at an early age of 'junk' foods. This may sound slightly 'earth motherish' and unkind, but think of it in the long term: what the eye doesn't see, the heart doesn't grieve over! They will need less dental treatment and will have less fat on their bodies. Fat children get tormented terribly at school and their size is usually not their fault but that of their parents. And fat children usually grow into fat adults!

Talking of body fat, it is worth mentioning Nigel Benn, the British boxer who had such a low percentage of body fat that he began feeling quite unwell. It was only when he had a medical check up that doctors found his fat percentage dangerously low at 5.5 per cent. I hasten to add that this is not likely to happen to the majority of us, but do be aware of what could happen if you cut down on certain foods too drastically. The important thing is not to become paranoid about your weight. You have to retain a good balanced diet which contains a healthy mixture of carbohydrates, fats, proteins, vitamins and minerals.

SWEETENERS
If you down a lot of diet drinks or put artificial sweeteners in your tea and coffee, you are not really doing yourself any favours, because you are keeping your taste buds tuned to a high level of sweetness. Your palate doesn't differentiate between artificial and natural sweeteners – it just tastes sweetness, and it gets used to the level at which you feed it. So if you're trying to lose weight on lots of artificially sweetened cups of coffee, apples and Diet Cokes, your taste buds – all 10,000 of them – are constantly screaming for something sweet and it becomes almost impossible to get rid of the desire to take in more sweet food than you need. Hence the odd binges on chocolate, cakes, etc.

Therefore, if you want to lose weight, don't waste money on alternatives, just cut out sweeteners. This sounds easier said than done (it is) but really, it's the only way. The first thing you have to do is to reduce your intake of both sugar and sweeteners, and gradually cut them out completely. You will almost certainly experience withdrawal symptoms such as headaches and rattiness, and will generally become a pain in the neck, but as long as you realize this is part and parcel of the end result you crave for, you will be able to cope – just warn everyone around you of what you are doing and ask for their help and support!

JUNK FOODS
Our working bodies could be compared to fires or stoves: if they are not fuelled properly, they will die down. If you burn a pile of paper, it whooshes up quickly and then peters out to a pile of dust. If you add something more solid to the fire, it lasts longer. It's the same with our bodies: if we fill them full of junk or 'incorrect' food, we get a rush of energy almost immediately but then the energy level drops and we begin to feel lethargic and hungry again. If we feed ourselves something more

substantial, such as fresh raw fruit and vegetables, the energy level will rise steadily and will stay high for longer.

Junk food is invariably incredibly heavy in fat. Fat is stored in the body in a layer which lies over the muscles and just beneath the skin. If fat is not used up as energy in some sort of activity where you sweat and burn up calories, this is where you will store the excess. Just think of fat intake being stored in the body as fat. So, as a chocolate bar is high in fat, it will be stored somewhere within the fatty layer. Obviously, it will melt down a bit in the system and spread itself around, slowly easing itself into all the little nooks and crannies where it manifests itself as flab; and unless it is used up as energy, it will stay put!

HOW NOT TO LOSE WEIGHT

When eventually you realize there is too much flab hanging around and you begin to see bulges where your knickers end beneath tight skirts or trousers – the VPL (visible panty line) or YFL (Y-front line) – you may decide to go on a crash diet, skipping a few meals and drinking a few more black coffees. This seems to be the obvious solution; you've convinced yourself that now is the time to lose weight and reckon you might as well do it quickly before your incentive disappears. However, dieting in this way is disastrous.

When you drink coffee, your stomach fills with liquid. The toxins such as caffeine have to be filtered out by the kidneys which have to work overtime for the purpose. Your body then pees away the most important part – water, which, as noted above, is a vital part of your body make-up. And if you diet by black coffee and starvation, you're asking for trouble both physically and mentally! Drinking coffee and tea when you have hunger pangs is crazy. Caffeine, which is present in coffee, is a drug – you may notice the 'high' or 'buzz' you get from drinking a cup or two. I react like this, and have had to reduce my intake drastically as I have become caffeine-sensitive. This is a false boost of short-lived energy and when the effect has worn off you will feel lethargic and low. If you are a 'one cup a day or every other day' person, you may notice how hyped up you become almost instantly after drinking a cup. Your system is sensitive to the drug caffeine and your resistance to it is relatively low. This is somewhat similar to the 'buzz' smokers have after smoking the first cigarette of the day. When this energy wears off, you have a 'refill', and this is when your level of expectation rises and to hoist your energy level up from the depths to which starvation has reduced it you constantly turn to the coffee pot – often simply from habit (remember the guinea pigs' diet sheets!). If you don't move around enough to rid your body of this instant energy, the blood vessels around the heart have to work harder and the pulse rate increases. You should therefore never drink coffee before exercising as it can 'hype' you up too much, tempting you to push yourself past your safe limit. This is one reason why you should get into the habit of taking your pulse when exercising to keep a check on yourself.

It should be clear from this that coffee and starvation is the worst diet route you can take. You'll feel awful, you'll have no real energy, and if you go on and lose weight too quickly, you'll probably be left with stretch marks, making your skin look like a well-used ice-skating rink. And once you've got stretch marks, you're stuck with them!

Don't be fooled into drinking tea as a coffee substitute though; this also has a high caffeine content, as well as tannin. Take a look at the inside of a teapot and see how well stained that may have become. Now think of your own insides! Try to opt for natural infusions instead: these can be bought in most chemists and health food stores. The safest bet is just to drink water or diluted juices; try hot water with a slice of lemon. But, given recent news about the state of the country's water supplies, it wouldn't be a bad idea to go for bottled water instead of taking it straight from the tap! If you do drink tap water, take care with water filters, though: not the jug type of filter but the sort that is fitted directly to the mains water pipes. It seems the latter actually harbours germs and bacteria. In fact, in an article in the *Sunday Times* (22 October 1989), we are told that 'Water filters being used in thousands of British households to purify tap water can cause contamination and pose a health risk'. This is because the filters actually catch and absorb particles from the mains water supply, and when those particles and bacteria accumulate in the filter, they multiply. Some of the suppliers of filters recommend changing every three years; health experts feel they should be changed at least once a month, and in Canada the government has actually considered banning this type of water filter. Draw your own conclusions!

THE RIGHT WAY TO LOSE WEIGHT

If you want to lose weight, as mentioned previously, it has to be lost gradually. If you lose too much too quickly it will go from the wrong tissues: not from the fatty layer you are trying to get rid of, but from the muscles. This process is called 'ketosis', which means draining energy from the muscles instead of taking it from the body's fat stores. So by dieting too drastically you literally cannibalise your own flesh. Eventually, the muscles suffer, becoming weaker while the fat still sits enveloping your body, bold as brass and refusing to budge.

My programme works on both the fat – which it will shift – and the muscles – which it will tone up. The two layers should be thought of as being quite separate. Fat does not turn to muscle, nor does muscle turn to fat. This idea is a complete fallacy resting on a misunderstanding of our anatomy. Think in basic terms: the skeleton is covered by muscle, the muscle is covered by fat, and the fat is covered by skin. This isn't very technical and as you can see, the three layers are quite different.

Try not to lose more than 2½ lb in weight each week. Much more than this, and your fat store will be retained while, as mentioned previously, you 'eat your own meat' – not a pretty thought! Remember that it is within the fatty layer that your cellulite problem is, if you have one; it is there, not in your muscles, that you have those lumps and bumps that must be got rid of, and you can only do that if you diet properly – i.e. gradually and healthily, and exercising as you go.

Losing too much weight too rapidly is a disaster in the long term: you'll be left with hanging loose skin and quite possibly, more than your fair share of stretch marks, where skin once stretched over your excess hasn't been given time to 'shrink' back. Stretch marks are actually little scars and cannot be removed with creams or lotions. (You can help them fade to a certain extent, though, by rubbing in Vitamin E oil. This will take them from an angry red to a silver glow!) Also, slimmers who lose a tremendous amount of weight over a short period of time and don't exercise are usually left with a lot of hanging flab. Obviously this can be covered with clothing, but when they look at themselves naked and see hanging flesh, they become depressed and turn back towards food (usually the wrong sort) as a 'comforter'. This type of weight reduction then becomes a big psychological battle because although the slimmer knows that eating the wrong food will put back the flab at a rate of knots, it somehow doesn't seem to register in the mood of depression: it is almost as if by bingeing they are destroying their self-image, punishing their bodies for being in such bad shape. I had one client who noticed that while her legs were becoming firmer her stomach was taking too long to tone up – so she ate two huge tubs of ice cream and then became increasingly depressed because she had 'pleats', as she called them, on her midriff, where the flab hung in folds. Ice cream seems to be a favourite 'binge' food, perhaps because it is an obvious 'no no' and also perhaps because we can remember how good it was to be given as a treat in childhood. Perhaps, as mentioned previously, if our treats had been in the form of fruit, we wouldn't now have the problem of stuffing ourselves with 'empty calories' every time we felt slightly depressed. I wish I'd known this from an early age because I find it very difficult to pass by the confectionery counters when I feel cheesed off and force myself towards the fruit instead. However, every now and then I still need chocolate, usually just before a period when I crave something sweet. If this happens to you, go for black chocolate as this at least provides a certain amount of iron, which is what your body is really craving; but ration it – don't scoff the whole lot!

Trying to get toned up can seem like being trapped in a 'Catch 22' situation. To be firm and reduce body fat, you have to enjoy your regime. If you don't, you won't get anywhere. But if you're used to turning to all the wrong foods and drinks for pleasure, you'll have to change your habits – or you still won't get anywhere! Cut down on junk foods gradually and be aware of your body constantly. The following are all junk foods on which you should try to cut down drastically (but not all at once; if you know they are definitely 'out' you'll crave them even more and probably go on a binge): cakes, especially those with cream, fresh or otherwise; biscuits; snacks (crisps, salted nuts, etc.); jams/conserves; hamburgers/hot dogs; confectionery; colas; and virtually anything from a take-away where you can buy 'fast food'. If you really do want a 'take-away', opt for soup (read on and you'll see why). Look at this list and you probably think that all the joy in life has been taken away in one fell swoop; but then take a look at all the excess flab you want to rid yourself of!

Cutting out certain foods is going to give you quicker results, but you're going to have to dig deep to find your willpower. If you want lasting results and at the same time want to eat well, prepare your own food. This doesn't take too much time, just a little organization.

I recently had to have an operation on my tongue and couldn't eat anything 'solid' for a week and a half because of the stitches and general discomfort; I couldn't chew and was afraid that if I did, I'd bite my tongue! But I still had to go out to clients and teach: this meant that although anything I ate had to be pulverized so that it was soft, it also had to be very nutritious. I didn't want to eat tinned food as I needed my vitamins and minerals and didn't need all that salt and sugar; I knew that if I prepared my own 'mushy' food, I would be getting just those nutrients I wanted in some shape or form. I began my day by eating pulverized fruit or lukewarm porridge (everything had to be either cold or lukewarm and easy to eat): I needed something substantial inside to provide energy and to start the day. I then lived on home-made soups and juices; the recipes were easy and quick (they had to be, as my life was very hectic) and all used pulses or fresh vegetables. These usually came via a mad dash to Portobello Road (literally, to avoid the wheel clamps): I wanted them fresh, not sweating in plastic from the local supermarket. Some of the soups (gazpacho, for instance) retained vegetables in their raw state, and others were only lightly cooked.

In a week I lost just over half a stone, and this was without trying – purely through necessity. Obviously, I'm not suggesting you do the same otherwise I'd be contradicting myself; for the best results you have to lose weight gradually, as I have explained previously. Here I am just trying to make the point that you can lose weight by eating wholesome fresh food, which should include pulses, potatoes, grains and rice – just cut down on the fat! I could have lost less weight if I'd included wholemeal bread, but this was obviously impossible because I couldn't chew!

So diet gradually and sensibly and be sure to get your daily requirement of vitamins and minerals; eat plenty of fresh fruit and vegetables. You shouldn't need to take supplementary vitamins in the form of pills.

There is a risk of getting into a rut while dieting, and it's easy to suffer from depression. This is an emotion which will have to be taken into account when you seriously decide to embark on your regime. Remember, as with anything worthwhile, a health and fitness programme takes time and you will probably have to re-educate your whole way of thinking – gradually! Try to keep your mind active when on a diet; it's easy to stray off the rails and become bored. It doesn't have to be hell to be healthy!

If you think your motivation might need bolstering from time to time, get a good, discreet friend to take a 'before' photograph of your heavy parts (but be sure to keep the negative yourself, and keep it securely!). If the fat is all around your bottom and the tops of your legs, flex these areas so that you can see the fatty ripples! Or you can try taking a Polaroid of yourself standing between two mirrors, which means you don't have to bare all to anyone else. Keep a copy of the print (again, securely) in your diary or wallet and whenever you make a lunch date or are tempted to binge, you will see the blobs you are working to rid yourself of. One of my clients did this, and also kept a tarantula in a bottle in the fridge. The two strategies together worked wonders!

You must take care, though, to reach a happy medium, i.e. a suitable exercise programme and healthy eating regime that doesn't encourage anorexia (hardly eating at all) or bulimia (eating and vomiting), conditions which can easily develop if you become obsessive about diet and weight. Anorexics emit a slightly 'acrid' smell. This is because they eat away at their muscles, using protein for energy instead of fat stores. I have come across people with anorexia and bulimia who try to disguise the smell with garlic, mothballs and heavy perfume!

METABOLISM

Exercise will certainly increase your metabolism and you should notice yourself having to go to the loo far more frequently once you get going on your programme.

The more sluggishly and slowly a person moves about, the more their body will want to retain toxins and the slower their metabolism becomes. They need to go to the loo less often than a more active person with a faster metabolic rate and will probably revert to pills and powders to 'help them along' – a very unhealthy attitude!

I know of a chap whose only exercise was counting his millions and cleaning his teeth. He had a very high cholesterol level and thought that by cutting out cheese and chocolates from his diet, he would revert back to his youthful healthiness. The problem was that he was in his early fifties and because of his general lack of exercise had to take powders every morning to 'keep himself regular'. Instead of walking he would drive – 'much more civilized', and 'what was the point of having a good car if you were going to walk?' Poor chap, he could have been so much more interesting; but his energy level was low, his sex drive was zilch and he was nurturing a good spare tyre. After a day of meetings he would fall exhausted in front of the television set – what a ball of fun!

The body tends to retain fluid and toxins if it is allowed to, but there are ways of reducing these – exercise, massage and a healthy diet. If you feed your body regularly with junk and processed food, your metabolism slows down as your gut becomes lazy. This is because it isn't being fed enough fibre or roughage, which is found in cereals, raw fruit and vegetables (there is no fibre in fish, meat, eggs, juice, milk, alcoholic drinks, or sugar). One client developed diverticulosis apparently due to eating a diet of mainly processed food over the years.

CONVENIENCE FOODS

In processed and junk foods, nutrients are reduced during heating and freezing. There also tend to be many additives, such as salt, sugar and the dreaded 'E' numbers, and the fat content is usually extremely high to make the food more palatable. The nutrients which our bodies desperately need to absorb in their natural state are reduced during processing and even more with reheating.

As a nation of fast workers, we tend to reach for convenience foods a lot. In the mornings we're usually busy getting ourselves ready for work or hauling the children off to school, and we generally tend to lead hectic work and social lives. We invariably use our brains more than our bodies in the office and more often than not, the quickest and easiest way to prepare a meal is to pop something into the microwave. Obviously, this is a brilliant way of feeding ourselves more or less instantly when we feel famished and exhausted but our choice of food usually leaves a lot to be desired.

Remember, if something pre-packed is only going to take a couple of minutes to heat up, it has probably been mass cooked initially, reducing vitamins and minerals. It has then perhaps been frozen, when it loses even more, and by the time you heat it again the nutrients have probably waved goodbye and been blasted to pieces and you're left with a plate of sloppy fatty stodge – yummy! So do think carefully before buying convenience foods. Try to use them only in an emergency and try to get into the habit of keeping only one packet in store at any time. (Let's face it, most of us couldn't survive without them.) If you have to resort to using them, try to add something raw such as a side salad which can be bought ready prepared from the supermarket; these are ideal if you eat alone and they should last a couple of days in the fridge (but no longer).

Or eat tomatoes, which should only be cut immediately prior to eating to retain the vitamin level. Obviously, the sooner raw vegetables are eaten, the higher the vitamin content.

As a simple guideline to basic healthy eating, get into the habit of reading the ingredients on food labels. The higher up the list an ingredient is, the higher the proportion of it in the food. Take the following random examples:

HOVIS WHEATGERM: Unbleached wheat flour, water, cooked wheat-germ, yeast, salt, vinegar, dextrose, emulsifier E472(e), soya flour, flour improvers: L-ascorbic acid (vitamin C), 924.

Notice how high up the list salt is – 1.5 g per five slices. When I spoke to British Bakeries, I was told 'this is what the consumer likes'! The daily salt intake recommended by the Health Education Authority is 1 g; so with just five slices per day, you've had more than your 'recommended' allowance of salt!

SAINSBURY'S SAVOURY RICE: Rice, salt, sugar, dextrose, turmeric, hydrolysed vegetable protein, hydrogenated vegetable oil, dried onions, spices, dried garlic, dried mushrooms, parsley.

As you can see, salt is again very high up on the list. In fact, this tasted so salty I actually couldn't eat it and had to dispose of it, but perhaps this was just my own personal taste. However, on the list of ingredients, the salt content is listed as being 1.5 g; again, well over the recommended total daily intake. When I wrote to Sainsbury, I was told that my letter would be brought to the attention of the Nutrition Labelling Committee who will investigate this particular product. I presume the investigation is still continuing as they didn't reply.

MARKS & SPENCER TAGLIATELLE: Cooked pasta (semolina, water, egg and spinach), milk, ham, chicken stock, mushrooms, cream, Parmesan, medium fat hard cheese, margarine, wheatflour, modified starch, lemon juice, vegetable bouillon, salt, gelling agent, gelatine, pepper, herbs (less than 10% meat).

The salt content is 0.9 g and as you can see, salt is coming from all directions – chicken stock, Parmesan and 'solo'. M & S replied to my letter by saying that although they acknowledged the need to keep salt to a minimum, it would in fact continue to be widely used in order to offer the "most authentic and popular recipe" for each product.

So do start reading labels carefully. Remember, salt can 'hype' you up and will retain fluid. Excess sugar turns to fat in the body and sugars are empty calories!

If you feel a product is too salty or sweet, do contact the manufacturer and let them know your views. (For example, salt was omitted from Appleford's Cluster Bar after I wrote to them and we discussed salt contents. I was most impressed!) If the manufacturers get no 'feedback' (sorry for the pun), they will do nothing about remedying the situation. If we, the consumers, voice our opinions, they will quite possibly alter the recipe. After all, it's we who either enjoy or suffer a product and if manufacturers are not informed, how are they to know which it is?

3
PREPARING
FOR ACTION

LIFESTYLES

'I used to be 7½ stone' is a classic comment I hear when visiting clients for the first time. They seem so ashamed that they are hitting 9 stone or more which is more or less my own weight. Looks are deceptive. I'm petite but solid; it's just that I look lighter! This is because I exercise on a regular basis – I have to, and it is hard work – eat a good diet and have a regular massage. (If I don't have time to go to a masseuse, I pummel my own bits – see chapter 5 for a simple but effective self-massage routine.) What some of us forget is that those days when we were lighter are probably 5, 10, 15 or more years ago now, a time when we were probably much more active. If you are constantly rushing around, perhaps in a job where the adrenalin surges out constantly due to pressures of work, you are bound to burn up more calories. As soon as you move to a less active job, while you will probably be eating the same amount you will burn up less energy (calories).

Think of animals in the wild. They are more often than not much leaner and more active when they are free and can run around, and have to look after themselves. As soon as they are put into captivity, they become fatter and more lethargic. The less they do in the form of physical activity, the less they want to do and the more bored they become. Take a look at caged animals and see how frustrated they seem to be, facing the same scenery and the same dreary space day after day. They also seem to suffer from many stress-related diseases usually associated with boredom and lack of movement. Their only exercise is in pacing up and down, becoming still more frustrated. It's the same for us: the same routines, same workplace, same faces. Obviously, if you don't have some sort of variety in your routine you are heading for boredom and depression. This can affect your sex drive; and when this goes, everything goes. This is usually the time when we turn to a comforter, be it bingeing, boozing or smoking.

Activity, then, plays an important part in keeping us alert, both mentally and physically, with the added advantage of reducing fat mass and improving muscle tone.

BODY SHAPES

Body shapes have a lot to do with the distribution and storage of fat. As with our genes, some of us are more prone to storing fat in the form of cellulite than others. It literally depends on how our genes deal with the storage of water in fat. Basically, there are three types of body shape.

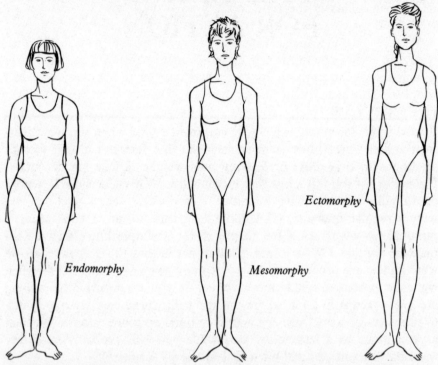

Ectomorphy

Endomorphy

Mesomorphy

Endomorphy. This is the typical 'pear' shape, usually small-breasted and wide-hipped. People who have this shape are usually short-limbed and have a tendency towards being 'stocky'. They have a high proportion of body fat compared to muscle. Endomorphs need to watch their diet carefully and exercise hard and regularly to keep in good shape. Because of their high fat density, which could be used as an energy storehouse, they do have 'staying power'. They usually do well at endurance sports, such as swimming and even long-distance running, rather than activities such as sprinting which use short, fast bursts of energy. People with this body type often find running longer distances much more of a struggle at the outset. However, endurance training must always be built up gradually, and if they have the willpower, they could make good long-distance runners.

Mesomorphy. This 'average' shape gives the impression of being 'petite'. Body fat is evenly dispersed. Mesomorphs usually have strong shoulders and arms and a tendency towards well-developed calf-muscles which can look quite shapely. They are good at most sports especially those which demand bursts of energy such as sprinting, tennis, squash and a few team games. Take a look at the short-distance runners on the television: they tend to be well developed and strong. With a good diet and regular exercise, this body could become the perfect shape.

Ectomorphy. This is the type of body most of us would give our eye teeth for: long and lean with legs 'up to the armpits'. Height can help to foster a general elegance. However, many tall people tend to feel self-conscious about their height; the worst thing they can do is stoop or slouch in the attempt to hide it. Ectomorphs rarely have a weight problem. However, if they don't exercise, they could reach middle age with rather small, saggy bottoms and hanging loose flesh which may make them look rather droopy! Sometimes women with this shape have trouble in childbirth, as the pelvis usually tends to be quite narrow.

Whatever your shape, you are in danger of suffering from the 'floppy syndrome' – flabby stomach, thighs and bottoms – if you don't participate in a good exercise regime. The flab really manifests itself when you reach your forties. One day you reach the big four-O and the next day the flab appears: and it gradually gets worse. When flesh hangs loosely, it is ageing and unsightly and there are limitations on just how much can be covered up!

HOW DO YOU KNOW IF YOU'RE OVERWEIGHT?

In my research, I purposely didn't use skin calipers to measure fat loss because I thought this would encourage readers of my book to go out and buy them, and unless you are expertly trained and have a hundred pounds plus to spare on a good set (the cheaper versions tend not to be too reliable in an amateur's hands), you could be both getting incorrect readings and increasing the bank charges on your overdraft! Also, forget the old saying of 'if you can pinch an inch' around the waist you're overweight. Even the slimmest of us can pinch an inch or two, or more!

A more reliable and simpler test to find out if you're carrying excess weight is to buckle up a belt around the lower part of your ribs and slide it down to your waist. If it doesn't budge, you're carrying too much flab. Obviously, if you're pregnant it won't budge at all, but then, this programme isn't designed for you: you should read my *Prenatal Exercise Handbook* instead!

Some people carry excess weight on their stomachs, some on their bottoms and others on their legs, and some have it everywhere. So just see if you have an odd handful of looseness anywhere that wobbles when you move. If you do, and you feel 'sluggish' and lethargic, go by that and get to work on yourself!

Perhaps you should try on one of last year's outfits which you looked so good in. If it fits but you feel flabby, you just need to tone up. If it pulls out of all proportion, you've become fatter, and need to reduce. Watch your diet and get cracking on some exercise. But remember, there is no way you can 'spot' reduce with diets: if anyone says you can, they are talking out of the back of their neck! You can't swallow food with instructions 'avoid the stomach, legs etc.'; it just doesn't work! If it did, I'd have a much smaller bum by now.

Take a look, too, at the height and weight chart on page 43. But remember, it's firmness and fitness you're aiming for, and the tape measure is just as important as the scales – if not more!

When you diet, fat loss will go from the heaviest parts first. The excess around your middle, that is, the waist and hip area, will be the first to shift, followed by that on the bottom and tops of the legs. It is important to exercise at this time, otherwise you'll have the 'hanging flesh' syndrome.

BOTTOMS

There seem to be two particular types of bottom which are somewhat unattractive: those that are as flat as a pancake and droop, and those which are so wobbly they can be compared to two people struggling beneath the sheets trying to get out, shaking and gyrating in all directions. I looked around at the shape of behinds, on both men and women, in different areas of London. The wobbliest bottoms in the metropolitan area seem to accumulate in Richmond and Twickenham, and the droopiest in Kensington and Knightsbridge (probably due to too much sitting). The flattest tend to shuffle around the West End and the widest in the East End. Whether there is something in the water or what, I really don't know, but the amount of wobbling flesh in those parts of the city is amazing!

Sagging bottoms can creep up on us all, men as well as girls. The first thing I notice on a man are his eyes, the second, his toupé (I prefer a bald man any day!), the third his brain and the fourth, his bottom (unless he is facing the other way, in which case, read in reverse order!). Men can become so unattractive if they have a sagging bum. So girls, don't think you are the only ones this book is aimed at: men should follow the regime too. Take a look at your partner's *derrière*; does it honestly come up to your own high standards? Is it firm and approachable or loose and floppy? If the latter, make him read this with you! Men tend to develop beer bellies and loose bottoms, while women have a leaning towards droopy bottoms, floppy thighs and loose stomachs; but neither need be the case any more!

Some of the largest muscles in the body are in the bottom (some much larger than others), the *gluteus maximus* and *gluteus medius*. You can see from the diagram how the muscles entwine. Different cultures produce different shapes. Take, for example, the West Indian and African races. The majority of both men and women tend to be overweight, a result as much of dietary as of hereditary factors. However, they tend to have beautifully rounded and usually very firm bums and thighs and a wonderful sense of rhythm: when they move, and even more when they dance, every movement seems to stem from the bottom! Watch 'Merengue' or 'Lambada' dancing – tight yet fluid movements which use all the muscles in the upper leg and bottom. Orientals, on the other hand, tend to have extremely flat and low-slung bottoms. Take a look at most orientals sideways on in tight skirts or trousers and you will usually notice very little definition between the back and the front, with very little curvature on their bottoms. Of course, this is hereditary. South Americans have a word for such rear ends: '*Culiplancha*', which literally translated means 'flat-bottomed'.

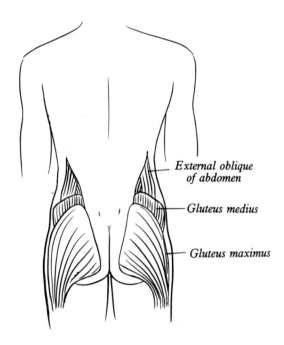

External oblique of abdomen

Gluteus medius

Gluteus maximus

Europeans tend to have a mixture of both the above shapes, usually not too big or too small although there are the odd exceptions – I'm one of them! I seem to have an 'African'-shaped bum and can actually balance a glass on it while still standing – a good party trick if the conversation lapses – it's like a shelf! I don't know where it was inherited from, all my sisters have the 'normal' versions. Usually, Europeans tend to carry more width than depth. I think the character of the British has a great deal to do with how we move. We tend to be very reserved as a nation. The more introvert a person is, the more likely he or she is to have a loose, shapeless bottom, basically, I think, because people like this want to hide everything, including their behinds, and what is not seen isn't worth worrying about!

Or is it? If the muscles in your bottom sag, you can count on muscles elsewhere doing the same, given time: gravity loves to pull them down. So what do you do? Stand on your head for twelve hours a day? Nothing quite so drastic – but if you intend firming up your bottom you are going to have to work hard. However, if you set your mind to it, nothing should deter you and you should, with regular practice, notice definite results within six weeks. If you don't work regularly, you won't! Therefore, if you've been planning a holiday on the beach where you will be wearing little or no clothing, and are worried about your shape from the waist down, now is the time to get started – don't leave it a moment longer or you will feel like staying under wraps for the duration of your vacation, especially when you notice the younger, firmer, sylph-like creatures appearing in front of your eyes and those of your partner!

BACKS

Many of my students, especially the men, have been put off working on their abdominals because of bad backs. Backs are precious and have to be handled with care. If they are treated badly, they will react badly. There are three main skeletal defects to which backs are subject. If you have any one of these, you must take care while carrying out your abdominal exercises as your positioning may have to be varied slightly. Again, do check with your GP beforehand. Show him or her this book and ask if there are any exercises which should be avoided in your particular case.

Lordosis. People with 'lordosis' – sway backs – can be ideal candidates for straining the small of the back (lumbar region), which is a classic area for back injuries. This is because the 'hollow', the small of the back, tightens and takes the strain when you do any form of lifting. Whenever you stand, make sure you tilt the pelvis backwards i.e. tuck your bottom under to elongate the back, which in turn lengthens and stretches the muscles along the spine. I write first hand about Lordosis as I have this particular curvature.

Kyphosis. In this phenomenon the middle of the spine tends to bend backwards with the pelvis pushed forwards. This can give a slightly concave appearance to the chest area and a very round-shouldered effect.

Scholiosis. This is a lateral (sideways) curvature to the spine which can happen anywhere down its length.

All the above defects have to be taken into account when performing abdominal exercises. If you have any of them, take care. But though your positioning may have to be adjusted slightly, you should still be able to work at the abdominals and have rippling muscles the same as everyone else!

MEASUREMENTS

Before you start your programme, make a note of your measurements, and update this over a six-week period. *Measure in centimetres* once each week on the same day: don't put it off, and you keep an accurate record.

The measurements in the table were taken from Joanne during her six-week trial.

| | Week no. | | | | | |
	1	2	3	4	5	6
	Centimetres					
Wrist	18	18	18	18	18	18
Upper arm	39	37	36	36	35	34
Chest	100	98	97	96	95	94
Waist	90	86	85	84	83	80
Hips	116	112	110	105	103	99
Tops of thighs	69	67	66	64	63	60
Calves	48	47	46	44	43	40

As you can see, weight goes from the bulkiest parts first. Jo is still working on her programme and is still losing centimetres. She now eats sensibly and has much more energy.

BONE SIZE

To determine bone size (frame size), take your wrist measurement on the bone.

Women

Small frame	5½" (14 cm) or less
Medium frame —	5½–6" (14–15.2 cm)
Large frame	6" (15.2 cm) or more

Men

Small frame	6¼" (15.8 cm) or less
Medium frame	6¼–7" (15.8–17.7 cm)
Large frame	7" (17.7 cm) or more

You may be pleasantly surprised or mildly shocked by this gem of information. Or maybe you will realize you can no longer get away with the excuse 'I'm big boned, that's why I'm so heavy'.

HEIGHT AND WEIGHT
Check your height as well as your weight. If you exercise on a regular basis, you may become as much as an inch taller, by stretching the muscles and improving the posture. With this regular workout therefore, you have a 'package' deal. You lessen the fat/cellulite percentage, tone up the muscles and stretch a little.

The height and weight chart reproduced on page 43 was devised by the Look After Yourself Project at the Health Education Authority and shows what is considered the acceptable weight range for your height and sex as well as the level at which obesity begins.

CHECKING YOUR PULSE RATE
So you realize that you've been overindulging a bit and that a few bulges have appeared which you have been tenderly nurturing; and you decide to heave yourself into an exercise programme to achieve rapid results.

If you have been inactive for any length of time or work at a sedentary job, it is important that you take it gradually and monitor your progress. I'm sure you've all heard of people going on to a squash court or running a marathon and dying of a heart attack. This is because they pushed the body into doing more than it was actually capable of. It is important therefore, if you haven't participated in any form of physical activity for some time, to build up your efforts gradually and to get into the habit of checking your pulse or 'heart rate'.

In this programme you will be putting pressure on the large muscle groups, primarily those in the legs. The metabolic rate has to be increased and to do this, you must make the muscles in the legs and bottom work hard. It is also advisable to monitor your heart rate to ensure you don't work into a 'danger' zone by pushing yourself beyond your physically safe level.

Checking the heart rate is relatively easy. Place your first three fingertips (not your thumb as the skin on the fingertips is more sensitive) on your pulse. You can find the pulse either in your neck – to the side of your Adam's apple – or on the inside of your wrist. Follow the line of your thumb down to its base and place your fingers just below the wrist bone. Count the beats you feel in 15 seconds and multiply by four to give you a one minute reading. Start with the figure zero and then count. You will get a more accurate figure if you time yourself using a non-digital watch or clock. This is because with a digital clock you may be tempted to count seconds by the markings on the clock rather than the beats of your heart. If you find it difficult to concentrate, ask a friend to check your time for you.

Height & Weight Chart (LAY Project, Health Education Authority)

MEN: weight without clothes

Height without shoes		Acceptable average		Acceptable weight range				Obese	
m	ft in	kg	st lb	kg (low)	st-lb (low)	st-lb (high)	kg (high)	kg	st lb
1.45	4- 9								
1.48	4-10								
1.50	4-11								
1.52	5- 0								
1.54	5- 1								
1.56	5- 1¼								
1.58	5- 2	55.8	8-11	51	8- 0	10- 1	64	77	12- 1
1.60	5- 2¾	57.6	9- 1	52	8- 2	10- 3	65	78	12- 4
1.62	5- 3½	58.6	9- 3	53	8- 5	10- 5	66	79	12- 6
1.64	5- 4½	59.6	9- 5	54	8- 7	10- 7	67	80	12- 8
1.66	5- 5¼	60.6	9- 7	55	8- 9	10-12	69	83	13- 1
1.68	5- 6	61.7	9-10	56	8-11	11- 2	71	85	13- 5
1.70	5- 6¾	63.5	10- 0	58	9- 2	11- 7	73	88	13-12
1.72	5- 7½	65.0	10- 3	59	9- 4	11- 9	74	89	14- 0
1.74	5- 8¼	66.5	10- 6	60	9- 6	11-11	75	90	14- 2
1.76	5- 9	68.0	10-10	62	9-10	12- 1	77	92	14- 6
1.78	5-10	69.4	10-13	64	10- 1	12- 6	79	95	14-11
1.80	5-10¾	71.0	11- 2	65	10- 3	12- 8	80	96	15- 1
1.82	5-11½	72.6	11- 6	66	10- 5	12-12	82	98	15- 6
1.84	6- ¼	74.2	11- 9	67	10- 7	13- 3	84	101	15-12
1.86	6- 1	75.8	11-13	69	10-12	13- 7	86	103	16- 3
1.88	6- 1¾	77.6	12- 3	71	11- 2	13-12	88	106	16- 9
1.90	6- 2½	79.3	12- 6	73	11- 7	14- 2	90	108	17- 0
1.92	6- 3¼	81.0	12-10	75	11-11	14- 9	93	112	17- 8

WOMEN: weight without clothes

Height without shoes		Acceptable average		Acceptable weight range				Obese	
m	ft in	kg	st lb	kg (low)	st-lb (low)	st-lb (high)	kg (high)	kg	st lb
1.45	4- 9	46.0	7- 3	42	6- 8	8- 5	53	64	10- 1
1.48	4-10	46.5	7- 4	42	6- 8	8- 7	54	65	10- 3
1.50	4-11	47.0	7- 5	43	6-11	8- 9	55	66	10- 5
1.52	5- 0	48.5	7- 9	44	6-13	8-13	57	68	10-10
1.54	5- 1	49.5	7-10	44	6-13	9- 2	58	70	11- 0
1.56	5- 1¼	50.4	7-13	45	7- 1	9- 2	58	70	11- 0
1.58	5- 2	51.3	8- 1	46	7- 3	9- 4	59		
1.60	5- 2¾	52.6	8- 4	48	7- 8	9- 6	61	73	11- 7
1.62	5- 3½	54.0	8- 7	49	7-10	9-10	62		
1.64	5- 4½	55.4	8-10	50	7-12	10- 1	64	77	12- 1
1.66	5- 5¼	56.8	8-13	51	8- 0	10- 3	65	78	12- 4
1.68	5- 6	58.1	9- 2	52	8- 2	10- 5	66	79	12- 6
1.70	5- 6¾	60.0	9- 6	53	8- 5	10- 7	67	80	12- 8
1.72	5- 7½	61.3	9- 9	55	8- 9	10-12	69	83	13- 1
1.74	5- 8¼	62.6	9-12	56	8-11	11- 0	70	84	13- 3
1.76	5- 9	64.0	10- 1	58	9- 2	11- 4	72	86	13- 7
1.78	5-10	65.3	10- 4	59	9- 4	11- 9	74	89	14- 0

To find out the minimum and maximum pulse rate you are working to, complete the following simple equation (supplied by the Health Education Authority)

200 minus age   =⎫
200 minus age minus 20   =⎬ Upper range
200 minus age minus 40   =⎭ Lower range

The top of the upper range is the absolute maximum you should push yourself to and the bottom of the lower range is the minimum you should aim for. Take, for example a 40-year-old:

200 minus 40   = 160⎫
200 minus 40 minus 20   = 140⎬ Upper range
200 minus 40 minus 40   = 120⎭ Lower range

And a 35-year-old:-

200 minus 35   = 165⎫
200 minus 35 minus 20   = 145⎬ Upper range
200 minus 35 minus 40   = 125⎭ Lower range

and so on.

RESTING PULSE

Take your pulse before you begin your exercise session to ascertain your 'resting' pulse. Take it again immediately after the aerobic section to see how hard you have pushed yourself and yet again after a further 90 seconds have lapsed to find out how quick your recovery rate is and to see how long it takes you to revert back to your 'resting' state. The quicker you return to your resting pulse, the fitter you are. Keep moving gently while you take your pulse after vigorous exercise to prevent 'pooling' of lactic acids in the muscles (to prevent the muscles becoming stiff).

To start off your exercise routine you should do an aerobic-type exercise of your choice (step test (see chapter 4), skipping, trampolining, jogging, cycling) for 15 *minutes*; anything less than this will not sufficiently raise the pulse and more does not proportionately increase benefits although it will prove you have 'staying' power! Obviously, in the beginning you may only be able to start with 5 minutes; this is perfectly OK but you'll have to build up the time gradually for noticeable results. After finishing your aerobic exercise take the pulse for 15 seconds and multiply it by four to get your reading. The 40-year-old should at least be within the 120–140 beats a minute range and should aim for no more than 160 beats per minute maximum.

A good rule of thumb is to work and talk, e.g. carry on a conversation or sing along with a record that you like to work out to. If you can't do either of these while working, you're overdoing it and should stop. You're obviously working too hard too soon!

You may think pulse monitoring is a waste of time. But think again of the sudden fatalities which just occasionally happen during exercising, and I think you'll agree it's well worth the trouble!

GETTING GOING – AND KEEPING GOING

If you really do want to get into shape and rid your body of fatty deposits it's going to take time and you can't go about it in a half-hearted way. Perseverance has to be a key issue. It's so easy to skip a day, or two or three, which then become a week, and so on. You have to decide that you're going to stay with the programme right from the outset. If you're a career person and don't think you'll get round to exercising after a heavy day, try getting up an hour earlier. There are no short cuts and I'm afraid you simply have to make time. Everyone has just one crack of the whip in this life and if you take a course which is going to make you unhappy, overweight and bored, heading for an early exit, you can more often than not blame yourself. However, if you choose to improve your lifestyle and get yourself into some sort of fitness programme, you'll have more confidence and much more enthusiasm. If, to reach your goal, you have to get up earlier, isn't it worth it? Besides, if you work at your programme first thing in the morning, you really will feel much more lively and energetic to face the day. Or you might try to work at your programme during the lunch break – just a thought for the enthusiastic! It doesn't matter when you do it, but do it!

Once you get into a regular pattern and start noticing the changes in your body shape, you will have some incentive to carry on. However, it will take approximately six weeks of regular exercise to produce a noticeable increase in firmness. Again, don't believe all these promises of instant results or results in a few hours; they're just not true. If you do, you'll probably push yourself too hard and end up injuring yourself by over-competitiveness!

Do get into the habit of checking your pulse as often as possible and in different situations; see how much it rises after an argument or when harassed. If this added release of adrenalin isn't used up in the form of physical exercise, the heart is ultimately taking the burden of excess stress and strain. Channel your energies wisely!

You will only get out of your programme what you put in to it! To get real results, you must try to work out for at least 45 minutes on six days a week: on the seventh you can mollycoddle yourself. However, once you get into the programme and notice the changes in yourself, you'll probably become 'hooked'! Initially, of course, the duration of your exercise programme will depend on your body structure and the actual fat deposit. Obviously, if you are grossly overweight, you certainly won't be able to keep going for a full 45 minutes, so build up gradually. Try brisk walking or swimming, just to get you started and to get you moving, and see how you get on. Gradually ease yourself into the programme. My research showed that weight loss and body toning were more effective if exercise was taken religiously for at least 45 minutes every day; taken out of 24 hours, it is not a lot to ask! Again, it all depends on how determined you are to get back into shape.

Also, if you are taking any form of medication or have recently suffered any illness or injury, or if you are very heavily overweight, this could affect your performance during a strenuous exercise programme and you should consult your doctor before embarking on this fitness regime. This is not, I hasten to add, because any of the exercises are controversial but merely to safeguard yourself from any possible problems.

Transformation won't happen just by thinking 'fit', it only happens with sweat and jolly hard work! One of the regulars in a club where I work has to change her leotard and adjust her make-up every time a little sweat appears. Forget it! You should be able to sweat buckets and forget your appearance. The idea is to tone up and not to worry about sweat marks. You can wash away sweat; you can't wash away flab!

4
YOUR EXERCISE PROGRAMME

THE AEROBIC PHASE

My clients started their programme off (after 5 minutes of loosening up) with an aerobic-type exercise, performed for at least 15 minutes. This ensured that the heart was beating strongly and the muscles were warmed for the remaining 30 minutes of the workout.

A lot of people still associate aerobic-type activity with prancing around in a slinky leotard. In my workouts, this isn't necessary. If they help, fine (like 'go faster' stripes on a car); but anything loose and comfortable will do.

Aerobic-type activity can be anything from brisk walking to cycling, mini-trampolining, jogging or dancing the 'Merengue' or 'Lambada' (Caribbean and South American dances); in fact any activity that raises the pulse rate and in which the large muscle groups are worked and have pressure put on them. I have purposely omitted swimming as this doesn't put enough weight on the legs, although it is a good way to exercise if you sustain injury at any time and can't do any of the other activities. To get maximum results, you have to put pressure on the big muscles and bones in the legs. If you have joint problems, mini-trampolining is your best bet for raising the heart rate. Using the large muscle groups ensures that a certain amount of 'loadbearing' is taken by the skeleton, which can help prevent osteoporosis – the breaking down of bone-tissue – in later life.

THE 'STEP TEST'

This is an extremely good way to get the pulse rate up and at the same time work the thigh and buttock muscles. You should work for 5 minutes if possible but if at any time you feel out of breath, dizzy or nauseous you must stop. The exercise is very simple: you literally step up and down. You can do this on your own stairs or alternatively on a low bench which should be approximately 13″ (33cm) high for women and 15½″ (40cm) high for men. Try not to hang on banisters etc.: make sure you use the muscles in your legs and not those in your arms to hoist yourself up. Obviously, if you're a short man, you'd use the shorter step and if you're a tall lady, you'd use the higher step. Usually, stepping up and down two stairs at a time is a good measure if you don't want to have a block specifically made. Sometimes we have to diversify and use what is to hand!

The leg you use to step up with is called the 'leading' leg. If you step up with the right leg followed by the left one, you should step down with your right leg followed by the left one. Change leading legs whenever you feel you need to but try not to lose momentum. Set your alarm for 5 minutes and when your time is up, stop, and take your pulse for 15 seconds, then multiply this number by four to find your heart rate. If however, you feel awful after only a few minutes (this can happen if you smoke, are asthmatic or if you are taking drugs of any sort), stop immediately and take your pulse. If you haven't reached your minimum heart rate, you've got a lot of work to do, and you'll have to work up much more gradually.

THE EXERCISE

Some of the exercises that follow can be done with a partner, some you may prefer to do alone and in private. And apart from your daily 45-minute session, you can tense and isolate muscles in most situations – while zooming around on the school run, during top-level boardroom discussions, during an argument – even during lovemaking! Whatever you do and wherever you do it, good luck: you will notice the benefits sooner than you think.

Different bodies react in different ways to the same exercise. Quite a lot depends, for example, on how long your ligaments are, which determines how far you can stretch out. If you have short ligaments you will find it more difficult to touch your toes than a person with long ligaments – but it won't be impossible, by any means. It just takes time and perseverance. So you may have to modify your position in a lot of exercises to reach the desired muscles.

If you experience cramping in the muscles during any exercise, stop straight away, rest, and slap the affected area to increase the circulation. When you're ready to continue, carry on. On no account keep going through cramps, or indeed any other pain: this is your body's way of screaming out for oxygen for the muscles and begging you to stop. Listen to what your body is telling you, or you'll do more harm than good.

REPETITIONS AND SETS

Eight repetitions of any exercise are called a 'set'. Start off with one set (eight repetitions), then if that feels OK go up to two sets (sixteen repetitions), three sets (twenty-four repetitions) and so on. Remember that you must always work the same number of repetitions on each side – e.g. sixteen on the right leg, sixteen on the left leg – or you'll become lopsided. Never be tempted to do more on your stronger side – if you do it will become stronger and stronger and the other weaker and weaker.

WORKING WITH WEIGHTS

(W) alongside some of the exercises denotes those that can be performed with the addition of weights which will help improve your muscle tone faster.

The principle to remember with weights is that more repetitions with lighter weights will tone, while fewer repetitions with heavier weights will bulk up the muscles. I'm assuming you want to tone and streamline your outline, so will be working with relatively light weights. Obviously, if you do want to 'bulk' up, increase the poundage accordingly. I'm not going to introduce you to the kind of exercise machines body-builders use!

When you start working with weights, you must build up gradually: don't start with, say, 32 repetitions using several pounds or you may well suffer irreparable damage. Start with a few repetitions and a light weight – perhaps eight repetitions using 1 lb. If this feels comfortable, increase to sixteen repetitions. Once you are confident doing three sets with 1 lb, try one set with 2 lb and increase the repetitions as and when you are able. When you reach three sets with 2 lb, progress to 2 ½ lbs – and so on, working up *at your own pace*. Whatever you do, you must increase gradually and don't overdo it. Don't be too enthusiastic at the outset otherwise your limbs will scream out. If ever there is any strain you must stop immediately.

GETTING STARTED

To achieve the best results, you must first feel the muscles you will be working on. If you don't identify the right ones, you could carry out a tremendous number of repetitions without actually benefiting, then give up thoroughly disheartened when you notice no improvement. Therefore, before you get going on any sort of regime, you should make sure you are feeling the correct muscle group. The most basic exercise to learn is flexion and relaxation. Start off by feeling the muscles you'll be working in your bottom.

Sit on a chair and flex up the cheeks of your bottom without using the muscles in your stomach. Try to keep the hands totally relaxed. Tighten the muscles as hard as you possibly can and feel your body raise up at least half an inch as you tense and flex them (don't hold your breath; keep breathing normally). Once you have managed to isolate this group, you are ready to begin.

Now stand up and try the same exercise.

To make sure you are doing the exercise correctly, place a finger vertically between the cheeks of your bottom and tense up the muscles. Grip hard, feel your finger getting squashed. Or use a pencil and try to pulverize it. Alternatively, imagine someone or something that you honestly dislike; if you find this difficult to visualize, think of your poll tax demand, the telephone bill or a photo of someone who makes life difficult for you generally. Place your imaginary item between the cheeks of your bottom and try to pulverize it by squashing your buttocks together as hard as you possibly can. Feel the muscles flex and tighten up; this is how they should be when you exercise this particular muscle group. By tensing your buttocks in certain exercises, you will also protect your back as this will prevent you from lifting limbs too high and hollowing the small of the back.

Years ago, while I was still training, I was told that the best exercise to tighten up the bottom was to sit on the floor and 'scoot' from one side of the room to the other, rocking and moving from one buttock to another. Forget this one; all you will do is get splinters in your bum, carpet burns, or wear out your carpet. Your buttock muscles need to *work*, not just be rocked from side to side!

A good basic all-rounder which will start working straight away on your buttocks and thighs is to walk with feeling. Instead of taking every step with gyrating, loose, floppy flesh, tighten up the muscles in your legs and bottom. As you walk, flex the thigh and buttock muscles and stride out. If you move loosely, you'll feel like a slug. If you move with confidence and tightness, you'll have your body more in control. Think tight!

BOTTOM/HAMSTRINGS:

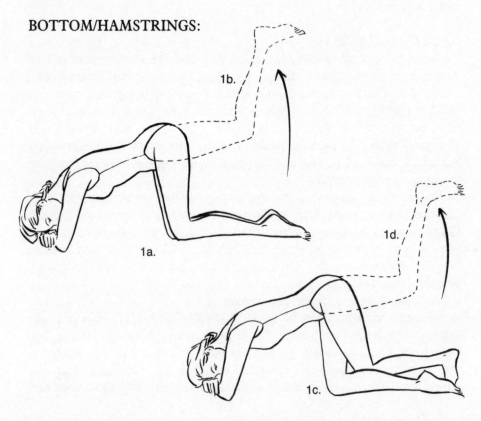

1. (1–5 sets) (a) Go down on to the hands and knees. Rest your forehead on your folded arms and keep looking down at the floor. This will protect the small of your back, reducing any tendency to hollow and strain it. (b) Raise one bent leg up towards the ceiling, (c) cross it over the other one, (d) bring it back up to position (b) and return to starting position. Make sure you centre your body; try not to lean towards the supporting knee which should remain squarely on the floor otherwise the supporting leg will take up too much strain and you won't exercise properly the muscles you are aiming at, i.e. those in your bottom. A progression of this is to carry on with the same exercise but instead of bending the working leg, keep it straight: you'll notice the thigh muscles working even harder! (W)

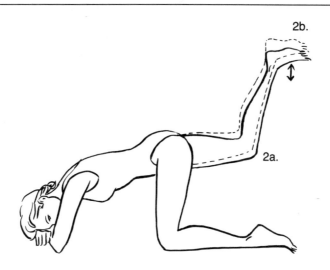

2. Stay in the same starting position as the previous exercise. Keeping the knees bent (as in 1b), lift one leg up as high as you can *without hollowing the back*. Then raise it a little higher to your limit. Lift until you 'feel' the muscles in your buttocks. Perform tiddly little raises and lowerings for 8 counts and increase to 40 (five sets) or more. Minute movements on the large muscles are extremely beneficial. (W)

3. Stay on your hands and knees but this time fully extend (straighten out) the leg. Again, perform tiddly little raises and lowerings for another eight counts. Be aware of your back: don't hollow it! If you feel you can, alternate eight bent leg raises with eight extended leg raises, gradually increasing the acts. (W)

You should now start to feel the muscles in your bottom waking up. When you have worked to your maximum number, stretch the leg out

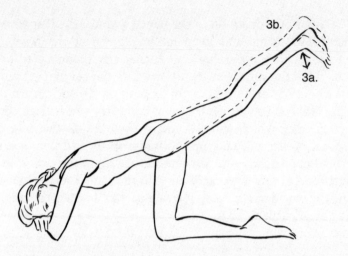

behind you on the floor and when you are ready, work the same number of repetitions on the other leg. If you find this exercise too hard on your knees, try the following alternative.

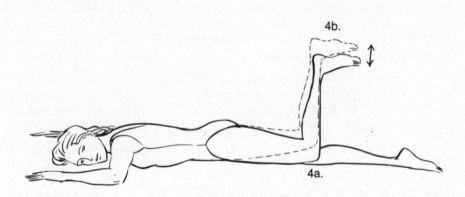

4. (1–5 or more sets) Lie on the floor on your front. Push the hips down into the floor hard. Keep the side of your face down on the floor, *not* resting on your hands. This prevents hollowing of the back. Bend one leg up while scrunching in the muscles in your bottom and thigh. Slowly raise and lower the bent leg as high as you comfortably can. If this feels OK, continue on to a straight (extended) leg lift. Again alternate bends with straight lifts, increasing sets. (W)

You should *never* raise or lower both legs together while lying on your back as this puts a tremendous strain on the small of the back (the lumbar region). You can, however, raise and lower them while lying on your front if you keep the hips and chest pressed down hard. The next exercise will firm up the bottom and strengthen the muscles in the small of your back: it has done wonders for one of my clients who broke his back in a riding accident – he now has much more strength, and is no longer harnessed up in the big, boned corset which he was wearing before his regime.

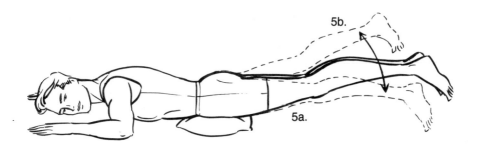

5. Lie flat on the floor, face down, pushing your hip bones downwards. (Men should place a pillow or small cushion beneath their hip area for obvious reasons – to protect their manhood!) It's imperative the hips stay down. If they don't, and you have a willing friend, ask her or him to push gently on your shoulders and buttocks to keep them down and to keep your back elongated. If there is any strain or if the hips still rise up, you should avoid this exercise altogether. Again, keep the side of your face down on the floor. Flex the muscles in your buttocks and backs of the thighs as hard as you can. (a) Slowly raise first one leg, then the other. Keeping both off the floor, (b) take them apart. Bring them back together and lower them slowly back down to the floor. Start with just one repetition. If this feels OK go on to two, then four and then eight. Rest in between sets of eight.

OUTER THIGH AND BOTTOM (ABDUCTORS AND GLUTES)

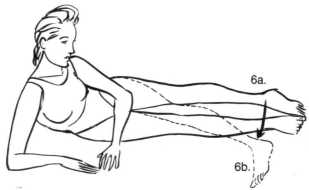

6. (a) Lie on your side with legs at a 90 degree angle (or as close as you can to it) to the body – an 'L' shape. (b) Raise the top leg, and keeping it straight, 'jump' it up and over, forwards towards your shoulders then

back towards the lower foot. Try to keep the top foot off the floor all the time and try to keep the toes pointing down towards the floor and the heel turned up towards the ceiling. Keep your arms in front of your body. Try 24 repetitions (three sets) and build up gradually to as many as you possibly can. Do the same amount on the other leg. (W)

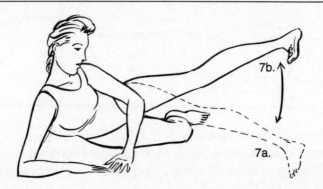

7. Stay on the side with the lower leg bent up towards the chest and both arms towards the front of the body. Bring the top leg out straight at a 45 degree angle. Aiming the toe towards the floor and the heel towards the ceiling, raise and lower the leg slowly. Try 16 repetitions and gradually increase in sets of eight.

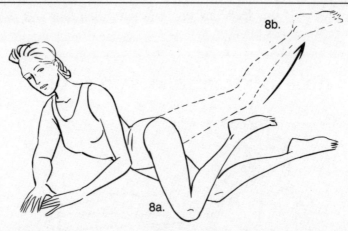

8. Stay virtually in the same position. This time though, cuddle up (a), dropping the top knee to the floor in front of the lower one. Try to keep the foot flexed and flat and aimed up towards the ceiling. (b) Gradually straighten the leg out and upwards, keeping the foot flat. Feel all the work in the buttock muscles and the hamstrings. Bend the knee back to the start position and carry on. Again, try 16 repetitions and increase in sets of eight.

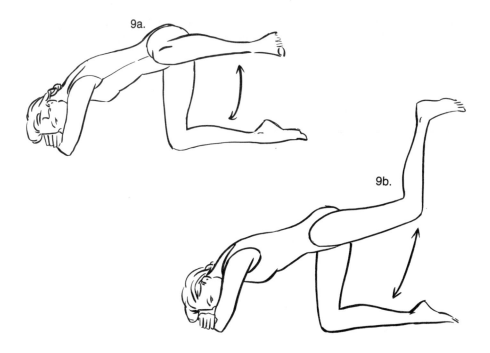

9. Go down on your hands and knees and rest your forehead on folded arms. Round your back to protect the lumbar region. (a) Raise one bent leg out to the side as high as you can, keeping the knee level with the foot (the raised leg should be parallel to the floor). Then lower it back down to the floor. (b) Now raise the foot backwards and up towards the ceiling. Don't hollow your back, and try to keep your weight centred: don't be tempted to lean too far over the supporting leg. (W)

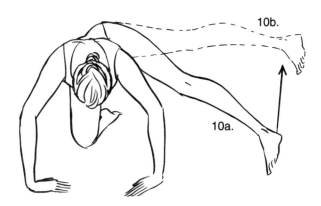

10. If you found the previous exercise too easy, progress on to sideways straight leg lift. Start in the same position, this time straighten the leg out to the side. Keep the toes turned down towards the floor and the heel

up towards the ceiling. Lift the leg. Again, try one set raising and lowering 3″ (8 cm) and increase gradually. (W)

All these exercises will give fantastic results on the saddle-bag area of your thighs and will definitely help lift up your bottom.

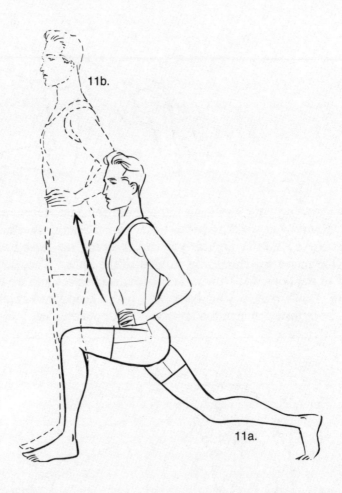

11. An excellent but fairly tough exercise for both legs and bottom is to go down (lunge) almost into a sprint position, but keeping the trunk up, and 'stride' out. Literally walk from one side of the room to the other in as low a position as possible moving forwards and keeping the back leg straight. Stand up between lunges. This will help firm up right around the thighs and bottom. (Be prepared for an aching bottom and tops of legs the following day though.)

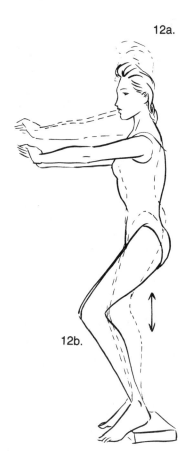

12. (a) Put a telephone directory on the floor. Stand with your heels on it, toes on the floor. Tuck your bottom under tightly and keep it under for the duration of the exercise. Keep your knees together and toes facing straight ahead (don't let them turn out), hands out in front to maintain balance, or on the hips. Slowly bend the knees, taking the strain in the tops of the thighs and in the bottom. (If you feel any strain in the knee joint, stop immediately – you're probably going down too far or are sticking out your bottom.) (b) Go as low as you comfortably can, then raise yourself back up using the muscles in your thighs. Start with one set and increase gradually. A progression of this exercise is to take the directory away and keep the feet flat on the floor. You must, however, still keep the bottom firmly tucked under, this will prevent you from going down too far.

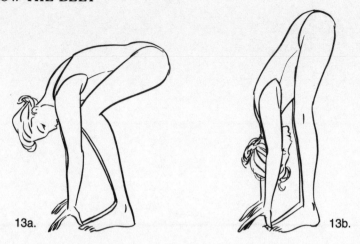

13a.   13b.

13. This exercise is an excellent 'all-rounder' for your legs. You must have at least your fingertips on the floor. By doing this you protect your back and only work the legs. If you bring your fingers off the floor you'll work into your back and could strain it. (a) Bend at the knees, keep your chest on the thighs throughout, hands on the floor and head loose. (b) Slowly straighten the knees as much as possible. The chest must remain on the thighs and fingertips at least must remain on the floor.

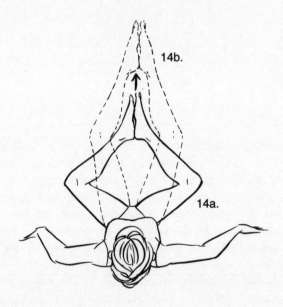

14b.

14a.

14. For the best results with this exercise, take your shoes off and keep the soles of your feet together throughout. Flex the muscles in your bottom while you work. (a) Lie on your back with your legs in the air

and knees bent outwards. Place the soles of your feet together. (b) Raise your legs up as high as you can, still keeping the soles of the feet together. Hold for a slow count of eight and release. Try one set. If you work properly, you should feel the muscles in the outer and inner thigh as well as those in the buttocks working.

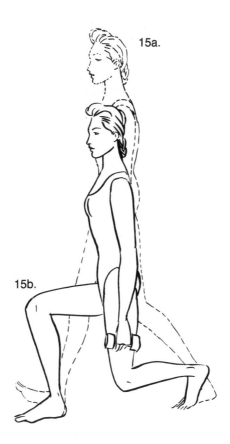

15a.

15b.

15. (a) Stand up and take one big step forwards. (b) Now bend both knees so that the back knee drops down towards the floor but not touching it and so that the front knee doesn't come in front of the toes. Use the muscles in the top of your thighs to push yourself up to the starting position. Once you can comfortably carry out two sets on each leg and if there is no strain on the knee joints, strap a weight to your wrist or hold a 'free' weight (1 lb to start, increasing gradually) and work up again from one set. (W)

LEGS

When your legs develop cellulite and the muscles become flabby, you've got a problem. You can cover up your bottom half to a certain degree during the winter months, but there will come a time in the summer when you want to expose your legs. Obviously you could live in long frocks and just hoist them up every time you want to brown your limbs in the sun; or you could wear long shorts. But this isn't much fun really, is it? And you'll probably end up with some odd suntan marks. So what's the alternative? The answer again is exercise – now!

The quadriceps – the big muscles at the front of the legs – take a lot of working on, as do the overhanging fleshy bits around the knees. Chubby legs and knees may look sweet on a toddler but most of us have outgrown that stage and this hanging, flabby and usually cellulite-ridden mass is just added extra baggage and depressing to look at!

One of my clients was flatly refusing to share a sailing holiday with her husband and friends because she was too embarrassed to bare her flabby thighs. It almost wrecked her marriage. She came to me in sheer desperation and we worked hard to get her legs back in shape. By the time the date came around, she felt firm and confident enough to go, and off she went. This is by no means a case of waving a magic wand. She had to work jolly hard and religiously used the weights.

A NOTE ABOUT KNEES

Remember when working with weights on your legs that your knees are precious and have to be treated kindly. If you have problem knees – you may have had trouble with cartilages or a touch of osteoarthritis – you still need to work the joints but must not strain them. I am kind to knees because I've suffered! Not through exercising, I hasten to add, but through an accident some twenty years ago, as a result of which I had to have a cartilage removed from my knee. The surgeon then decided to carry out a synovectomy – scraping out the synovial fluid which aids the smooth sliding motion of the kneecap. Years later this proved to be a great mistake and I suffered atrophy (wasting) of the quadriceps muscles and pain within the joint which has now become arthritic. To strengthen the muscle and get the tone back I had to carry out millions of repetitions of this next exercise. Work first without weights and then, when you feel able, with weights (light at first, as ever) on your ankles to help tone up even more.

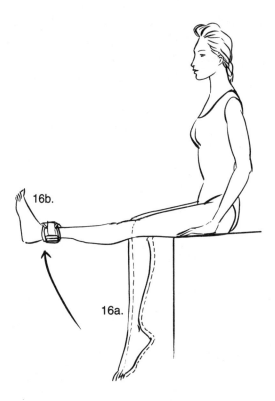

16. (a) Sit on a table or counter top or somewhere where your legs can dangle freely. Keep both cheeks of your rear firmly down on the surface. Flex the muscles in your thighs and flex your foot (don't point the toes or your may get cramp) – if you can't tell if you've flexed enough, put your hand lightly on your thigh and feel the muscles become harder. (b) Slowly straighten the leg up by pushing the knee downwards; hold for five seconds (don't jolt your leg up and don't drop it down – control it). Lower your leg back down slowly; repeat as many times as you comfortably can (at least two sets). Make sure you don't hold your breath, which is a common mistake. Do the same amount of repetitions on the other leg. Every day increase the number of repetitions. To make the exercise stronger, increase resistance by adding weights, starting with just 1 lb and working up to 4 lb or more on each leg. Don't use weights if you feel any strain in the knee joint. (W)

A progression of this exercise is to work from a standing position.

17. Bend the supporting leg very slightly, i.e. don't lock the knee joint. (a) Bend the working leg to 45 degrees and then (b) straighten it out, bend the knee back in, (c) turn it out to the side, rotating the hip, and (d) straighten it out sideways, keeping the knee as high as possible. Try

one set at first on each leg and work up to two or more. Again, add weights when you have reached at least three sets. With the addition of the weights, start with one set and again, increase gradually. (W)

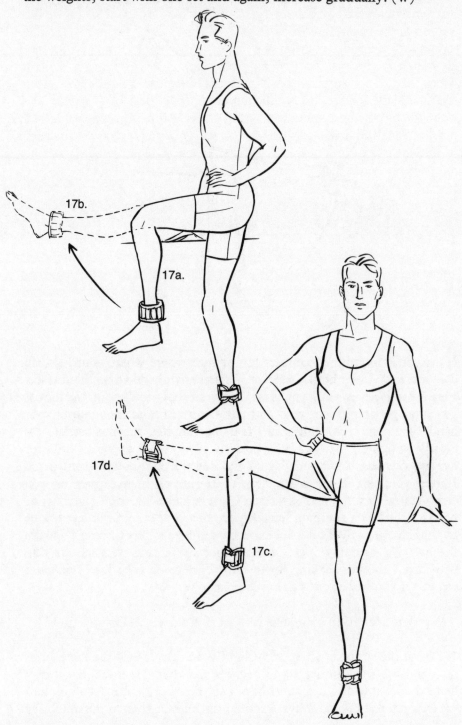

INNER THIGHS (ADDUCTORS)

The inner thigh is an important area to work on and one that can become extremely flabby as we get older. It's usually only when we get our bodies out on to the beach that we notice the hanging mass! You can frantically try to tuck it up into your knicker leg or bikini bottom but it won't stay: as soon as you move, out it will fall. Therefore you're going to have to work hard on a regular basis and use weights. These muscles are stubborn. We tend not to use them much, hence the flab. The fatty layer over the top of the muscle won't shift easily. However, exercising with lots of repetitions and regular massage should give good, noticeable results. It takes time, but don't get disheartened. That flab has probably taken years to get there and it won't disappear overnight!

18. Sit on the floor with your arms folded and your feet on the outside of two chair legs. Make sure your ankles are padded enough to avoid bruising i.e. wear socks. Gradually but firmly pull the legs in towards each other. Squeeze and hold for a slow count of eight and try to keep going for at least five sets. Initially you may not notice too much but after about three minutes of squeezing, you should notice the inner thigh muscles working. If you feel any strain in the knees at any time during this exercise, stop immediately.

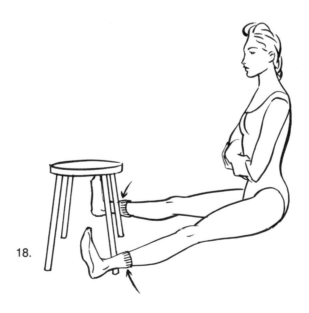

18.

19. (a) Lie on the floor on your side with the cheek of your right buttock down, straighten out the right leg with the toes pointing down towards the floor and the heel turned up towards the ceiling. Bend the left leg up, behind the right one with the toes on the floor and the heel off. Pull in the abdominals and flex the muscles in your bottom. (b) Slowly raise and lower the right leg. Try to lift the foot higher than the opposite knee. Feel the muscles on the inner thigh work. Start with eight repetitions and gradually build up to 32 or more, but remember, you're working on strength not endurance! Repeat the same amount on the other leg. Again, work against resistance. For quicker results, add your weights using 2lb initially and work up to 4lb or more. (W)

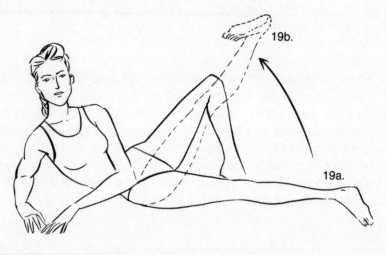

20. Still stay on your side on the floor. This time rest your top foot on a small stool about 18 in high. Keep both legs straight and pull in your tummy. Strap a 2 lb weight (to start with) on the lower leg, keep the inside of the foot facing the ceiling. Slowly raise the leg to meet the top one then take it slowly back down again to the floor. Try two sets at first and again increase upwards in groups of eight repetitions. (W)

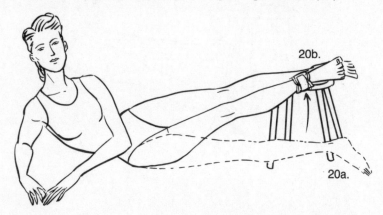

OUTER THIGHS (ABDUCTORS)

The outer thighs (abductors) are sometimes known as 'saddle-bags' – uncomplimentary but descriptive! You may see an extremely good likeness in a pair of old-fashioned riding jodhpurs – tight around the calves, big and bulky around the thighs! The saddle-bag area can become extremely floppy; it can, however (with a heck of a lot of effort), be whittled down and toned up.

This exercise might appear too easy at first, but it is effective – and the more repetitions you do, the harder it gets, so perseverance is of utmost importance. If you have a large mirror, wear a smile and nothing else, see the wrinkles of fat when you first start leg lifting and notice how they begin to disappear six weeks later.

21. Stand sideways on and hold on to a firm surface. Bend your inside (supporting) leg slightly i.e. don't lock the knee. Flex your outside (working) leg and lift it out to the side as high as you can then a little

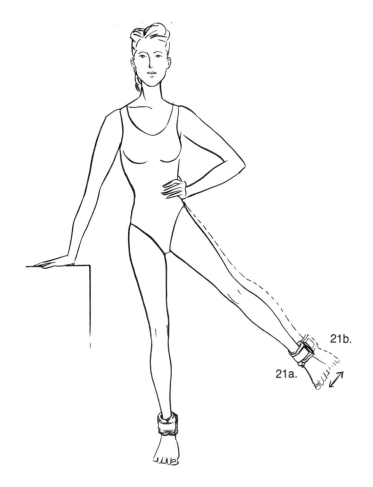

21b.

21a.

higher. Work up and down with tiny movements for a count of eight. Repeat the same amount for the other leg. Relax, and then try another set and so on. Again, once you can carry out four sets with ease do the exercise with 2 lb weights on your ankles, working up to 4lb or more on each leg. (W)

ABDOMINALS

It is essential to work the abdominal (tummy) muscles correctly to avoid putting excessive strain on those in the back. If you work incorrectly, not only can you actually 'distend' your stomach and look as if you're pregnant, but you may also end up with a permanent back injury. When working on abdominals – *abdominis transversalis* (upper) and *abdominis rectus* (lower) – your legs should either be elevated or the knees should be bent with the feet flat on the floor so that you force the small of your back downwards.

Initially you may find it difficult to isolate the upper and lower abdominals, but with practice you will get the hang of it. Men usually have the bulk of their bulge above the navel and women below, though there are exceptions! The following will work on both areas.

You don't necessarily have to carry out hundreds of repetitions of an exercise to benefit from it. If you do fifty or more and don't feel much, you're probably working on endurance rather than strength and certainly won't reap the rewards. I had one client who could do eighty stomach curls with no problem and with very little effect on her abdominals. It was only when I gave an alternative exercise to isolate the muscles more that she began to work the group I was aiming it; initially she could only manage eight repetitions. An exercise regime isn't just an endurance test: it's the results that matter. However, you shouldn't mollycoddle yourself while working on the abdominals. You won't get immediate results; no programme can offer this. If you've been inactive for months or even years, it's going to take time to bash the flab and get to the muscles, and you'll have to work jolly hard.

You should *never, never* either raise or lower both legs up off or down to the floor together while lying on your back. Nor should you attempt sit-ups with straight legs, as this will force your back to arch. Exercising in this way puts an abnormal strain on the lower back and again, you could sustain a permanent injury. Any instructor who ever asks you to exercise this way obviously doesn't know what he or she is doing and could only cause you long-term damage. Find another who doesn't!

The only exercise where both legs can be raised together is number 5 on page 53, where you are lying on your front; even here you must follow the instructions carefully.

To protect your back, you should first learn how to go about exercising your abdominal muscles properly. The next two exercises will help you feel the abdominals and you should always be aware of this 'tightness' while working on this particular muscle group. If the flexion goes while you are working on the abdominals, you should stop, otherwise your back will take the strain and 'bang', you'll pull a muscle which defeats the whole object.

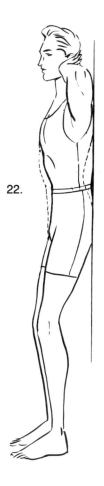

22.

Getting Started:

22. Stand up with your back against a wall with your feet about 4″ (10 cm) away from it. Bend your knees very slightly. Pull in your abdominals hard and gradually push the small (hollow) of your back into the wall. You may be very tempted to hold your breath and bring your shoulders up towards your ears, but *don't*! Try to relax the shoulders as much as possible and breathe normally. By tilting your pelvis backwards, you are elongating, as well as stretching and strengthening, the muscles in your back. This simple exercise will be invaluable.

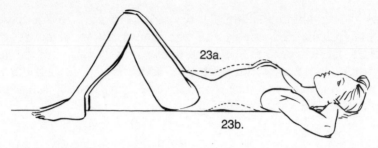

23a.

23b.

23. Another way to help isolate your abdominals is to lie on the floor on your back with your knees bent and your feet flat ('crook' lying). (a) Hollow up the small of your back and feel a gap between the floor and the lumber region (at the back of the waist). (b) Now, tilt your pelvis backwards so that you turn your pubic bone (and rude bits) up towards the ceiling. Push the small of your back downwards and pull the tummy in hard. You should feel the whole length of your spine flatten along the floor. If you are doing this correctly, the small of your back will be protected as the muscles elongate and become stronger.

Keep breathing and be aware of what is happening to the muscles around your middle. If you can't feel the muscles in your abdominals working, you're not pulling in hard enough. Keep practising. It's imperative that you master this before attempting the following exercises otherwise you could injure your back.

If you're still unsure as to whether you're 'tilting' correctly, ask a friend to put the fingers of one hand beneath the small of your back while you press down hard. If you squash their fingers, you're doing it right! *Keep breathing*; you don't need your stomach muscles to breathe, so don't hold your breath. When working on the abdominals, always tilt the pelvis backwards so that the pubic bone is thrust forwards.

With the following exercises, if you're very unfit start working with just one set of repetitions, work up to two and then more until you are doing as many as you comfortably can. Start gently, but don't be tempted to stop at one set every time. Remember, you have to work hard to get results! You will never make progress if you're half-hearted. Keep the momentum up and keep working!

24. Lie on the floor on your back with your knees bent. Put one hand behind your head and the other on your stomach area. (a) Push the small of the back down into the floor and keep looking up at the ceiling past your eyebrows. The hand behind your head is only being used as a support; on no account should you use it to 'yank' yourself up. (b) By pulling in the abdominals as hard as you possibly can, lift your head and shoulders off the floor, breathing out. As you lower yourself back down, breathe in. You should feel absolutely no strain in the neck, most of the

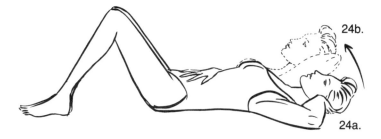

work is being carried out in the lower abdominals and you should actually feel them tighten up beneath your hand. When you know what you're supposed to feel, go on to the following exercise.

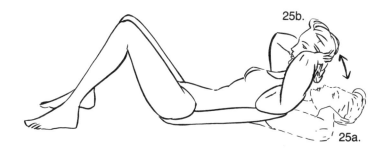

25. *Full trunk raises* (upper abdominals). Stay on your back with your knees bent, feet flat. Keep the fingers of both hands cupped or spread around your ears and the elbows wide. (a) Pull in the abdominals hard and raise yourself up as far as you comfortably can (breathing out) then lower yourself back down to the floor (breathing in). Start with one set of eight. It doesn't matter how far up you come, as long as you feel the abdominals work. Don't be tempted to 'jolt' yourself up.

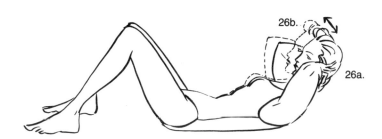

26. *Tiddly trunk raises.* Start in basically the same position as the previous exercise, but this time, keep your upper body off the floor until you've completed eight repetitions, raising and lowering yourself approximately 2–3″ (5–6 cms), then take a rest. When you feel relatively comfortable

with this, alternate the two exercises (25 and 26) i.e. eight full lifts off the floor and then eight tiddly ones from half-way. If you can manage three sets of each, you'll have a good abdominal definition in next to no time. Obviously, if you can do more, carry on; but be sure you're feeling the abdominals and not the neck and shoulders, which should be relaxed.

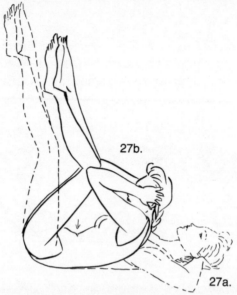

27. Stay on your back, raise your legs and cross your ankles with the knees bent. (a) Spread your hands around your head or cup your ears with your hands. Don't hold on to the gristly bits too hard or you'll feel as if your ears are about to be removed from your head! Don't clasp your hands behind your head either, otherwise you'll be tempted to use your shoulders and neck when lifting up. (b) Pull in the abdominals super hard and keeping your elbows out wide, bring your nose and knees towards each other, lifting your bottom off the floor slightly. As you take your legs away, extend them *up* towards the ceiling.

28. This time work both the abdominals and waist. Again, lie on your back with knees bent. (a) Cross one foot over the other bent knee and, keeping the top leg pushed outwards, pull in the abdominals hard. Put your hands around your ears and keep one elbow firmly on the floor (this will prevent you from 'yanking' up). (b) Flex the abdominals hard and bring the other elbow up towards the opposite knee, balancing on the support elbow and breathing out. As you go back down to the floor, breathe in. Keep going until you feel the stomach muscles working. You should feel no strain on either your neck or back; if you do, you're working incorrectly. Check that you are 'sucking in' the abdominals

hard enough. Begin with one set each side and increase the sets gradually.

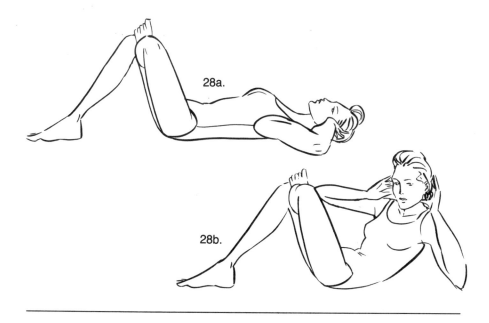

29. I call this exercise 'hotel room scrunches': it's what I recommend for my busy (or boozy) executive jet-setters who dash around the world on business trips, living out of suitcases and crawling from one heavy meeting to another. Stay on the floor and rest your feet on the seat of a sturdy chair, or better still, up on your bed. Make sure your feet are slightly higher than your knees. (a) Place one hand on the front of your thigh and put the other hand behind your head for support, keeping the

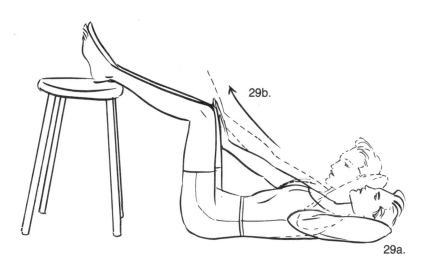

elbow out wide. (b) Tilt your pelvis backwards so that the whole of your back is on the floor. Bring your chin into your chest, scrunch in the abdominals hard and slowly pull yourself up while sliding the hand up towards your knees. It's imperative that you use the muscles in the stomach to lift and not those of your arms. You don't have to rise up very high, just far enough to feel the abdominals work. Start with at least three sets and increase repetitions at your own pace.

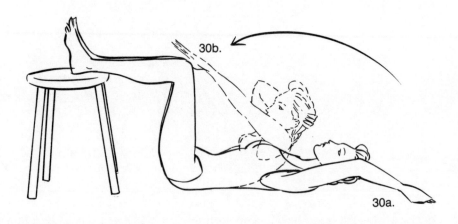

30. Stay in the same position. (a) Put one arm straight above your head on the floor and the other behind your head to support it. Pull in the stomach muscles tightly and again tilt the pelvis backwards. (b) Bring your chin towards your chest at the same time as bringing the straight arm up into the air and then down between the knees, lifting your upper body and breathing out. As you take the arm back down to the floor above your head when lowering yourself down, breathe in. By now you should really feel the abdominals working. Once you have got the hang of the above exercise and can comfortably carry out four sets, progress on to the advanced abdominal exercises.

ADVANCED ABDOMINAL EXERCISES

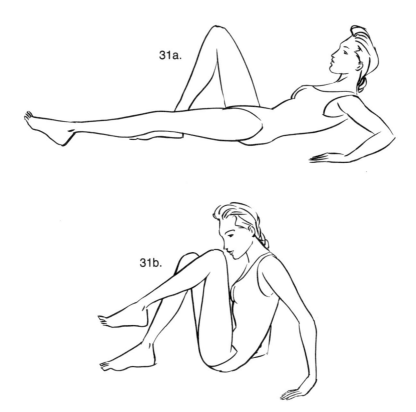

Lower Abdominals

31. Stay on the floor on your back. Bend one leg (a) keeping the foot flat on the floor. Straighten the other leg out and rest on your hands with fingers facing towards your bottom. Keep the elbows just off the floor and bent. Pull in the abdominals hard and keep the back rounded. Keep your chin tucked in towards your chest; breathe in. (b) Bring your knee up towards your nose at the same time as you push up, and straighten your elbows; breathe out. Start with one set and work up. With this exercise you have the added bonus of toning up the flabby underside of the upper arm as well as the legs and stomach!

32. Lie on your back with arms down by your sides and the head pressing firmly into the floor. Bend the knees up, keeping the feet off the floor. Pull in the abdominals hard and by pressing your arms and head and back down hard into the floor, bring your bent knees very slowly towards the chest, lifting your bottom gradually off the ground. Make sure all the work is being felt in the abdominal area. If you find this exercise easy, go on to 33.

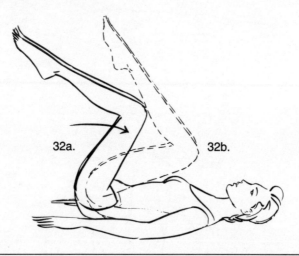

33. (a) Lie on your back with both legs up in the air. Keep your arms down by your sides and press both these and your head down hard into the floor. Pull in the abdominals hard and lift your legs up towards the

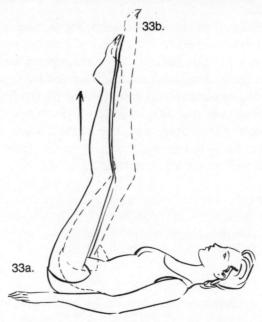

ceiling. (b) Lift your bottom off the floor as much as you comfortably can; don't bash your bottom back down to the floor, control it and lower it carefully. *Don't* try to take your legs behind your head as this puts strain on the back of the neck at the base of the skull. The toes should point skywards and *not* towards your head. The idea of the exercise is to isolate the abdominals totally.

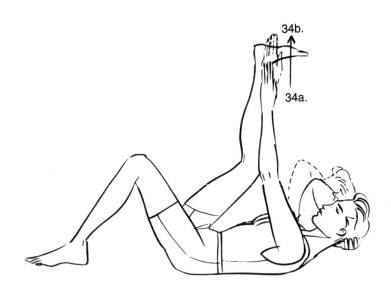

34. Lie on the floor in 'crook' position. Raise one leg up (it doesn't matter if the knee is bent). (a) Place one hand behind your head and bring the opposite hand to the raised leg up to the ankle bone. Pull in the abdominals hard. (b) Slowly slide the fingers up towards the instep and back down to the ankle bone. Make sure all the effort is in the abdominal area and not in the neck. Again, work in sets of eight. Try two sets on each leg and gradually increase.

Upper Abdominals
35. Stay down on the floor. Bend the right leg, keeping the foot flat on the floor, and straighten the left leg out to help anchor yourself. Hold on to the side of the bent knee, making sure your back is rounded. (a) Pull in the abdominals super hard and flex the muscles in your bottom. (b) Now let go of your knee, link your fingers and keep the elbows held out wide. (Keep breathing!) (b) Slowly turn to the left side and try to place your left elbow down towards the floor but not on it (don't be tempted to lean back). Just go as low as you comfortably can. Return to the starting

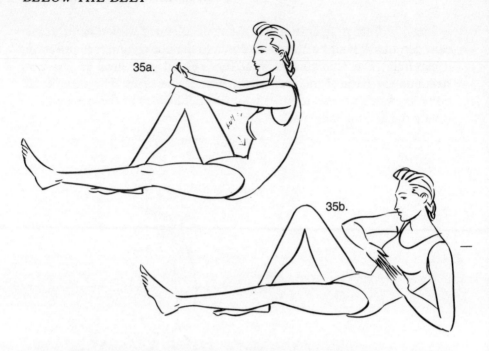

35a.

35b.

position and then turn to the other side. Try one each side to get the 'feel' of the exercise, then gradually increase repetitions. If there is any strain at any time on the back, stop immediately.

WAIST EXERCISES

This exercise will get rid of the flab and tone up the area around the waist, taking in all the overhang between the armpit and the 'love handles' – the area immediately below the belt and above the cheeks of the bottom!

Begin the exercise without weights and once you feel confident with how you're working, try holding a weight in the hanging hand. Begin with 2 lb and work up to whatever feels comfortable. Remember though, don't try too much too soon!

Stand with feet slightly wider than hip distance apart with the feet turning outwards and with the knees slightly bent, abdominals pulled in.

Keep the body facing forwards all the time i.e. on a lateral plane, don't be tempted to lean forward or backwards. The movement is sideways.

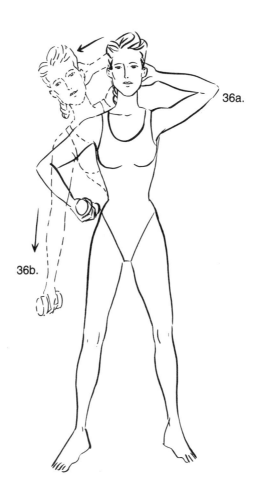

36. Start the exercise: (a) Place the fingers of your left hand on the left side of your head, keeping the elbow turned out. Bend the right elbow up with the palm towards the body. (b) In one fluid movement drop the right arm down which in turn will stretch the left elbow upwards. Return to the starting position and continue in sets of eight. Repeat but this time working the other side. For best results start with two sets. (W)

WAIST, STOMACH AND SIDE BULGES:

Go through this exercise slowly and when you feel confident, for the best results, use a light weight, say 1 lb to start with, increasing as you feel able.

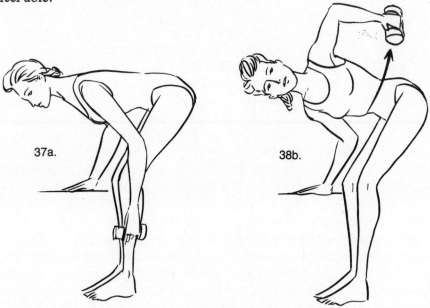

37a.   38b.

37. (a) Place your right hand on a low stool about 1 ft (31 cm) high and keep it there. Your left arm is straight and hanging down towards the floor. Place the feet just about hip distance apart with knees bent. Pull in the abdominals hard and keep the back as flat as possible. (b) In one movement, bring the left arm upwards forcing the elbow to bend and your body to rotate so that your chest is now turned towards the left side. Try eight repetitions and increase gradually, working the same amount on the other side. (W)

PELVIC FLOOR EXERCISES

This is, to me, perhaps the most important exercise section aimed specifically at women. It's more important to have strong pelvic floor muscles than a tight bottom or firm thighs. This exercise has the added advantage of improving your sex life and will actually stop embarrassing leakages.

You may be one of the unfortunate group who won't even attend an exercise class because you know you have a 'leakage' problem. You may have noticed this when you've had to run for the bus, when you've sneezed or even when you've had to lift something heavy. You will remember the embarrassment and sensation of shock when you felt your damp undies. You may even have to wear panty pads in your underwear continually because of weak pelvic floor muscles. Lots of women are too embarrassed even to consult their doctor about leakage, and so without help and guidance the situation worsens. But this problem is simply one of poor muscle tone, and there is no reason why it should continue. If you follow this really simple routine to strengthen and tone your pelvic floor muscles, you can only benefit and you don't even have to set aside time to work on them! With regular practice, you should notice a marked improvement. As ever, how quickly you get results depends entirely on how often you are prepared to work.

To test whether you have a problem, jump up and down on the spot for a few minutes, sneeze or have a good laugh. If you have any leakage/dampness, you've got weak pelvic floor muscles and these will only get worse if you don't get cracking and start working on them now.

Perhaps you've never heard of pelvic floors; most women haven't. They are usually only brought to your attention when you become pregnant and you're taught how to 'hold back' to prevent you from pushing and bearing down in the final stages of labour. So what happens if you never become pregnant? Why are we never taught about these muscles anyway? Maybe because they have something to do with 'rude bits' and a vast number of people still don't like to talk about 'private parts'. If they do, they usually use very technical terms and we are none the wiser. Or perhaps they don't know how to explain how they work, or don't even know they exist. There is still an awful lot of ignorance and naivety concerning this area. However, virtually nothing gets left out of my classes and this set of exercises is no exception: they are my forte – they are important! A huge number of women won't attend exercise classes for the simple reason that if they run, jump or even sneeze they end up with an embarrassing leakage and damp knickers. If only they had been told at an early age that the openings between their legs have to be exercised regularly as well as all the other bits in order to keep them strong and tight.

Basically, pelvic floor muscles are a group of muscles which lie at the bottom of the pelvis and support the pelvic organs, having a 'hammock' effect. There are three openings: from front to back, the urethra (where you pass urine), the vagina (where you discharge blood every time you have a period) and the anus (where you pass bulk waste). Each of the three openings is surrounded by a circular muscle which is called a 'sphincter'. This opens and closes an orifice (opening). To locate your pelvic floors, try to stop the flow of urine mid-stream; feel the muscles tighten and become slightly hard. These are the ones you will be working on. Only practice pulling up in this manner until you get the hang of how they work. Don't work this way on a regular basis as some doctors seem to think it may have an adverse affect on the kidneys.

Now that you have located the pelvic floors, you should try to exercise them on a regular basis. This will prevent 'dribbling' and also prevent emitting an unpleasant odour (you may not even be aware of this and your friends may feel too sensitive about telling you). It will definitely improve your sex life too. A friend's husband mentioned that after having their second child she would probably be very loose. He (being from New Zealand) was never one to beat about the bush with words and described slack pelvic floors in a woman as leading to an experience 'similar to dangling a worm in a well' (needless to say not very flattering to himself). His wife was determined that her sex life wasn't going to fly out of the window so she practised pelvic floor exercises regularly. Now she never has any leakage at all. Externally she is still out of shape but internally, she is tight and he is happy! Now she's slowly trying to get all the other bits back together but she had her priorities right and knew what she wanted to tackle first!

You can exercise the pelvic floor muscles any time – walking around, working at your desk, cooking, driving, putting your feet up. Just master the simple routine.

1. In your mind's eye, imagine there is a big flexible hollow polythene tube inserted in your vagina. By using your muscles you are going to stick the sides of the tube together flattening it from the base to the top. Begin by sealing the edge at the bottom of the tube together.

2. Imagine the tube. Pull the muscles inwards and upwards tighter and tighter. Work up in stages, go toward different levels using your muscle power.

3. As you pull up harder and harder, imagine you are gradually pulling the sides of the tube together until you reach the top.

4. Keep pulling upwards and inwards as hard as you possibly can. When you get to the top of the tube, try to seal together one corner. Keep pulling until you have sealed across the top and have flattened the tube completely. Only then release and relax the muscles. This is the full extent of the exercise that you have to aim for.

If you don't like working with tubes, let your mind wander in a different direction . . .

Imagine you are waiting for a public loo to become vacant. To be slightly inconspicuous, you wait by a taxi rank across the road. As you wait a gorgeous hunk, who you've felt attracted to for a long time, walks towards you and begins to chat. You decide you'd like to get to know him better and so, even though you keep one eye firmly on the loo, you become involved in conversation. However, your nerves begin to play havoc and suddenly you feel more desperate to have a pee. You pull your muscles in hard to save yourself!

All of a sudden you realize the curry you had the previous night is beginning to take its toll (it must have been the Vindaloo). You should never have tried it that hot; too late now! How embarrassing. You have to pull up and in harder than ever.

You can feel the cold sweat of panic. You carry on chatting normally, trying to stay cool, calm and collected.

You then realize that the tampon you inserted (you have a period too!) is starting to fall out. But your new-found future date is still chatting, absolutely oblivious to your dilemma and you exchange telephone numbers. You keep pulling in harder than ever to save your face.

Suddenly the loo becomes vacant and he departs, you dash over (keep pulling in). Heaven!

As luck would have it, no loo paper! You ferret around in your bag, you did have tissues somewhere. Luncheon vouchers, £50 notes, where are the tissues? – public loos, ugh! 'your kingdom for a tissue' – the tissues appear; – relief, happiness – let the muscles go, relax.

Again, this is the sort of enormous 'pull' you have to work at to have any lasting effect. With regular practice, you can do this exercise standing on your head, metaphorically speaking – in fact, in absolutely any position, and you don't need to hide away while you do it. Nobody need know what's going on. Just practise as much as you can – while hanging out the washing, during board meetings, talking on the telephone; anywhere, any time: even during an argument. Instead of flexing up your hands, flex up your pelvic floors! Keep at it: it's worth it in the long run.

DIFFERENT EXERCISE ACTIVITIES

There are so many types of exercises to choose from, it seems the whole world is our oyster; or is it? Team sports are great if you're keen on finding other participants to work with; or there are the regimes where you can work without having to rely on others, and that is what this book is all about. You can choose your time and place; the only must is that you work on a regular basis.

Professional sportsmen and women seem to be so incredibly firm and fit that you may decide to follow suit and take up their chosen activity because you've seen their fantastic bodies on the telly and you'd like to model yourself on your idol! But what exactly will it do for *you*?

ICE SKATING

'What about ice skating, will this firm up my legs, thighs and bottom?'
Ice skaters do tend to have good strong legs and bottoms and yet seem to
be very light on their feet. Just look at the performance of champion
skaters on the box: they move so gracefully and leap all over the place. A
brilliant sport and a brilliant choice if you happen to be young,
enthusiastic and good at getting up early in the mornings; otherwise
forget it! Prize skaters have to be up at the crack of dawn seven days a
week so that they can have the ice rink to themselves to improve their
technique.

Have you been to your local rink lately? I have; I was inquisitive to see
how this activity might score on a scale of one to ten. I think I'd rate it
about ½ for a novice! Firstly, the ice was crowded so all I could do was to
go round in circles. The younger kids don't take too kindly to geriatrics
and wanted me either to join their 'whiplash' or get off the ice. Always
open to a challenge, I took them on. I tried it once: never again! I was too
petrified to let go and even more petrified hanging on. But I hung on for
dear life watching my past appear rapidly before me. As I say, never
again. That was one activity I would recommend you steer away from
unless you really are young and eager with nerves of steel. If you have
these qualities, you will no doubt see extremely good results. For the
novice who tootles around the ice rink perhaps once a week, when the ice
is packed with other enthusiastic bodies, you will gain very little as far as
strength and firmness are concerned, although you will improve your
balance. This is because you are restricted as to how far and fast you can
move. Therefore if you decide to take up skating to help rid your body of
excess flab, you must be prepared to put in a great many hours.

HORSE RIDING

As with any professional sportsman or sportswoman whose chosen
activity demands rigorous training regimes, you will rarely see an excess
of flab on a serious rider, certainly not on the body parts that are used
most – in this case, the legs, bottom, shoulders and arms. This is one
sport where you virtually think with your legs and if you're riding at
anything other than absolute beginner level you need some pretty good
muscles to be at all effective; and riding at speed is fairly demanding on
wind power too. However, if you just sit up on top of a placid horse for
an hour a week you won't be doing much for your muscle tone; and you
might bear in mind too that modern stretch jodhpurs do little for the
appearance of anyone at all broad in the beam. In fact, it's largely
the shape of riding clothes that has given rise to the idea that riding
makes you broad in the beam: it doesn't, it's just that the rather heavy-

bottomed shape characteristic of so many British ladies is shown off to worst effect in tight, light jodhpurs! At least the old twill sort had some decent bagginess to hide in.

So unless you're going to take it up seriously, I wouldn't expect riding to do much for your exercise campaign – better perhaps to get fit to ride, rather than ride to get fit! After all, the other thing about jodhpurs is that they do show off excess saddlebags.

TENNIS

Take a look at professional tennis players: their muscle tone is fantastic, with a very low body fat ratio. This again is due to the hours and hours of training that go into their work to reach a physical peak, together with an extremely healthy diet. However professionals work out off the court as well as on it, and tennis alone will not tone you up unless you spend hours and hours playing. This is because there is a tremendous amount of stopping and starting, apologizing to the players on the next court and searching for your lost balls. So if you want to take up tennis as a leisure activity, fine, but you'll have to work out as well if you have a lot of flab to lose. Just notice how many loose bodies there are on the tennis courts, hidden under track suits: it's usually the 'after the game' activities, the socializing, that draws the crowds to tennis clubs. Also if you're not too good at it, you can fall over your feet, rip tendons and have the added bonus for getting tennis elbow! You'll also need an endless supply of frilly knickers (for the girls) and shorts with big pockets (for the boys).

WALKING

The only type of walking which will be of any benefit in burning off excess fat is brisk or power walking. It will tone up the muscles in your legs and bottom and will not strain your joints. If you decide to walk on a regular basis, you must invest in a pair of good shoes. However, it's no good thinking brisk walking is a quiet stroll around the shops, forget that. If you want to stroll, do so, but don't include this in your exercise programme. The only noticeable difference will be an aching back and a hole in your wallet! If you shuffle along window shopping, you may put in the mileage, but you are really not working your large muscle groups hard enough and you will not raise the heart rate, which is essential if you want to burn off calories and excess fat.

With brisk walking, you should try to feel the muscles in the buttocks and thighs working as much as possible. Try to flex the muscles as you walk. Again, work against resistance on the muscle groups. This way you need not go so far and you reap the benefits far more quickly.

However, don't walk your whole route 'flexed' up; you must give the muscles a break now and then. So start off flexing the muscles in your legs and buttocks hard and walk the distance of two well-spaced trees or lamp-posts; then slacken off the flexion in the muscles for the next two; and so on. Walk tight. However, you must keep the pace consistent. Keep the muscles guessing, but keep them working. You should make the effort to 'stride' out.

Initially, your limbs will ache, especially those in the calves, thighs and buttocks. Lazy muscles being woken up from their inactive state get tired quickly!

Try to get out of busy traffic. Go to your nearest park or perhaps the beach if you're lucky enough to be able to get there. Get fresh air into your lungs instead of carbon monoxide and cigarette smoke. You need to avoid obstacles and you need to keep up the momentum. Go by time and not by distance initially. Don't be too adventurous at the outset otherwise you'll end up hating this exercise.

Stride out for ten minutes, take your pulse to make sure you are within your safe range (see the section on checking your pulse in chapter 3) and then do a few stretching exercises while the muscles are warm and to prevent them tightening up. Stand on the edge of a stair or the kerb and gently drop your heels slightly lower than your toes to stretch out the back of the legs, especially the calf muscles (*gastrocnemius*). Gradually increase your walking time day by day.

Ten minutes may seem a little feeble for the more energetic among you, but we all have to start off somewhere and many readers of this book probably haven't exercised for years. You can all be catered for.

If you really do stride out in your walks, you can raise your pulse rate quite a lot and become quite sweaty; this is a good sign! An even better sign will be your increased physical firmness.

When you get up to fifteen minutes, work on distance. Vary your route to avoid boredom. Every time you go out, increase your stride and gradually increase the distance. Invest in a pedometer to save measuring the distance on the map with your dental floss (which is what one client of mine did). This can be a little unreliable, especially if you floss out your teeth and use the same piece to measure again!

CYCLING

To achieve the best results from cycling, an exercise bike is a must. 'Boring,' you may say, and I'd agree to a certain extent, but it's effective.

When you ride out in the streets and hurtle around Marble Arch, as I do, the traffic can become a nightmare. You breathe in volumes of exhaust fumes, knock over or try to avoid pedestrians who seem to be in a world of their own, and suffer abuse from jerks who seem to resent cyclists – especially taxi and truck drivers and fast-moving whizz-kids in convertibles! Even in the country you're at risk from motorists racing round blind corners, and huge lorries in country lanes. No, an exercise bike is safe. Put it in front of the telly or get yourself a music stand and read a good book from it. With an exercise bike you can keep to a constant pedalling pressure, which is a must for steady results, whereas in street cycling, you have to stop and start so much that your legs can't keep up the same pressure for long enough.

If you think that cycling will help tone up the abdominals, though, forget it, because it won't. To work the abdominal muscles you have to isolate them; so just think of cycling as an exercise to tone up the legs and increase the heart rate.

YOGA

I thought I'd try a yoga class to see if any of these exercises would be advantageous in burning off excess fat. 'Be at one with yourself,' the advert said so I thought I would. I quite fancied being able to stick my foot up behind my head and be at one with myself. I persevered, but became thoroughly despondent when I found I was competing with 'spiders' in the class, who could turn their bodies into contorted shapes and still look blank. Perhaps they were hiding their pain well, or maybe they really were mystical beings. However, this didn't work for me and by the end of the class I just felt cold and lost, still waiting for the energetic bits to begin so that I could notice my new 'being'. After a few sessions I definitely decided this wasn't going to get rid of any fat and besides, I found some of the exercises quite controversial. There were double leg lowerings and backward rolls, which put strain on the lower back and the base of the skull. In fact, at that time I had a call from a client's daughter to say she had just injured her neck in a yoga class trying to do a shoulder stand and could I help?

I decided yoga was definitely out!

One of the things that puts many people off a sustained training programme is the thought that they can't vary what they do, and that they will get bored. This needn't be the case at all: top up your exercise routine with brisk walking, skipping, mini-trampolining, cycling, or 'step testing'. Just keep moving, and try to keep working!

5
MASSAGE

Regular massage alongside your diet and exercise programme will help break down the fatty cellulite deposits. Massage alone is not very effective in this respect: but team it with serious exercise and a good balanced diet and it will have lasting effects.

You can either go to a qualified masseur/masseuse (but do check on their qualifications first or you could well end up wasting your time and money) or you can work on yourself. If you can't get to a masseuse on a regular basis, it's worth trying DIY massage, because one-offs just don't have any lasting effect. It's much more effective to pound away at yourself regularly than to go and lie on a masseur's couch once in a blue moon!

DIY MASSAGE

You should work for *at least* five minutes on each leg every day. It's not a huge chunk of time and the results will be extremely good as long as you don't let yourself skip a day here and there. You have to persevere, just as you do with your exercise! If you work on yourself after you get out of the bath or shower it will seem less of a chore. You probably already spend a couple of minutes after drying off rubbing in moisturiser, so take a little more time to massage your problem areas, perhaps with a little oil – it's well worth the effort. Massaging away all that cellulite and fatty tissue is bound to take time and perseverance, but think of the long-term results and don't lose heart!

You might find massaging your own body slightly tricky at first, but once you get the hang of it you will both enjoy it and start to notice the results. There are however a few basic guidelines you must follow:

1. Never rub over varicose veins.
2. Never rub over bruises.
3. Never rub over recently formed scar tissues.
4. Never work over broken skin.

If you're not sure whether a vein is varicosed or not, consult your doctor before you start.

Before massaging, remove any jewellery from your arms and hands.

At best it will be a nuisance, at worst you may scratch or bruise yourself. Also, either cut your nails short or at least make sure there are no rough edges – you don't want to end up covered in cuts and scratches!

When you rub your body, be aware of the feel of the fatty pockets beneath the skin and imagine them breaking down under your hands. This might feel uncomfortable initially, but with time you will become accustomed to the feeling as the lumps and bumps break down and disperse.

With practice you will learn what pressure best suits you. Deep massage can be very beneficial but you need to take care not to rub too deeply or too hard or bruising might occur. However, the harder you work, the more effective you will be in breaking down the fatty deposits: if you rub too softly, you will not notice any difference, and an over-soft touch can be extremely irritating. Experiment with different pressures until you find what suits you best and work at that pressure.

You may well notice that you can take stronger pressure on some days than on others. Women in particular often feel more sensitivity on their skin in the days just before their period. If this applies to you, just work for as long as you comfortably can. At this time, slow, sweeping circular movements on the abdomen can be very helpful in relieving that awful dragging feeling so many of us experience.

There are a few basic strokes you should learn.

1. EFFLUAGE
These are long, smooth strokes which are used to relax and prepare the area before stronger pressure is used.

Sit and rest your leg so that the ankle is higher than your hip bone. Place the palms face down on the area to be worked. Using an upward movement from the knee to the hip, stroke the thigh slowly but firmly using the palms of your hands, first on the upper thigh (quadriceps) and then on the underside of the thigh (hamstrings). Pull the skin up towards your trunk. Press firmly as you move your hands upwards, gently 'dragging' the skin.

Do this three times working with slightly more pressure each time.

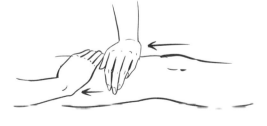

2. WRINGING

Wringing is carried out over 'fleshy' areas. Imagine you have a huge piece of very thick washing you wish to wring out, and so your fingers are spread, almost claw-like. This is how your hands should be for this particular 'stroke', so that you pull the flesh in two different directions. (Remember back to your school days when you gave Chinese Burns? This is the same movement.)

On your thighs you will be able to use your fingers to 'wring' by placing one hand alongside the other – fingers of one hand to the thumb of the other. Anchor your thumbs and pull the fingers on both hands out towards the thumbs. Work upwards from the knee to the thigh.

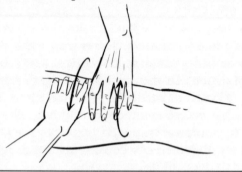

3. PULLING

This stroke can be used very effectively on both the inner and outer thigh areas. Again, the name says it all: you simply 'pull' the flesh firmly, using the fingers first of one hand, immediately followed by the other. Follow this stroke with 'kneading'.

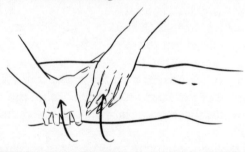

4. KNEADING

As the name implies, kneading is very similar to the movement used in bread-making. You literally knead your flesh. Push down with the thumbs and pull your flesh up with the fingers. This is probably one of the most effective strokes you will learn. You can actually feel the fat beneath your fingers and you can pull and push until you feel you've had enough. Pulling away at great handsful of flesh knowing that it is being pulverized is a very satisfying feeling. This will improve your circulation and break down fatty pockets beneath the skin's surface. It is a particularly good stroke to use on the inner and outer thighs, the insides of knees and the waist area where you can pummel away until your heart's content!

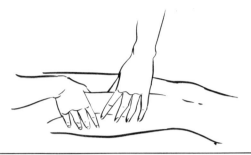

5. HACKING

With this stroke you use the side of your hands. Keep the fingers very loose and floppy and try to 'shake' them from the wrist. Again, this will improve the circulation. In the beginning your wrists may feel a little tired. However, your technique will improve with practice. Obviously, you will only be able to do this on the front of your thighs because of the angle you have to work at; but if you can educate a willing friend, you can have the backs of your legs worked on too.

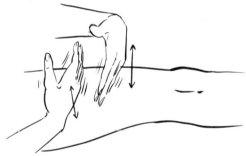

6. THUMBING

This is a movement I use a great deal. Hold the flesh with the fingers and thumbs, leaving a wide space between the thumb and first finger. Get a good hold. Press both thumbs into the fatty areas on the thighs and again, working from the knees up, use small circular movements to break down the fat.

7. KNUCKLING

If you can take 'thumbing', you can probably take 'knuckling'. Make your hands into a fist and use your knuckles in small rotating strokes to break down the fat. You may find this slightly more uncomfortable than the previous strokes, but if you can persevere, you'll find it extremely effective.

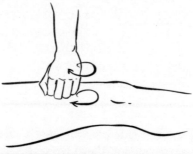

OILS

Once you have mastered the strokes, you may like to experiment with oils. Oils actually penetrate the skin and pass into the bloodstream, and will break down a certain number of fatty cells beneath the skin's surface.

Always work with caution when using aromatic oils, and don't use too much; if you do, you'll slip and slide over the skin's surface and you won't be able to pummel effectively.

You can either buy ready-made oils from a reputable source or you can mix your own. If you make your own, do stick to the 'recipe'; if the 'mix' is too strong you could experience adverse affects. However, with the right strength of the right oils you should notice a great difference in the general breakdown of your fat.

Oils which break down fatty tissues are juniper, fennel, rosemary, sage and lavender. Lavender is the most versatile of all the essential oils. It can be used in the treatment of cuts, burns, insomnia and nervous conditions. If ever you are in doubt as to which oil to use, you can always turn to this one. However, it probably isn't the best one to deal with the treatment of cellulite and in breaking down the fatty layer. The best 'mixture' I have found for this is a combination of 50 ml of a carrier oil such as almond (or, if your finances allow and you can find it, avocado – but this can be terribly expensive) with four drops of juniper and either eight drops of rosemary or sage or twelve drops of fennel.

Important: If you are *pregnant*, you must never use juniper, rosemary, sage or fennel oil. As a precautionary measure, only use lavender or vitamin E oil in your body massage.

If you have *high blood pressure*, never use rosemary oil.

If you are *epileptic*, never use sweet fennel, hyssop, sage or wormwood oils; again, you could revert to the ever-faithful lavender.

SKIN SCRUBBING

This is another good variation for breaking down fat and sounds far worse than it actually is. Soap a nail brush well and brush your skin while it's wet (until you get used to the sensation). This is one of the cheapest ways of improving the circulation and it really does assist in breaking down the pockets of fat beneath the skin's surface. Do remember, though, not to do this more than every other day for full effectiveness, and keep your skin well moisturized to prevent excessive dryness. When you are able to carry out skin scrubbing without gritting your teeth, progress to dry skin scrubbing. Before you get into your bath, dry rub your skin with either a loofah or a medium to hardish nail brush (if you can tolerate it); but only do this every other day for full effectiveness. If you over-stimulate the skin on a regular basis, the treatment will become less effective as you become almost immune to the feel of the scrubbing.

SALT RUBBING

Another good way of stimulating the circulation and thus helping rid the body of excess fat is to rub it with some form of crystals. These can be in the form of sea salt or Epsom salts. Stand in the bath and dampen your skin. Get a handful of crystals and rub them over the fatty areas. Work with rotating strokes and feel the skin 'come alive'. Shower it all off and then soak for a while in your bath. After you have dried yourself off, as with body scrubbing, rub in the oils which will help prevent the skin from becoming too dry and will penetrate through to the fatty layer.

LYMPH DRAINAGE

This is another form of massage, based on the lymph system. This one, however, can have side-effects, inducing headaches and vomiting; or you can feel totally relaxed. As the lymph is contained within its own system, it is more difficult to work on yourself. Therefore, lymph drainage is best left to a qualified masseur/masseuse.

6
WHAT ARE THE ALTERNATIVES?

PLASTIC SURGERY

LIPOSUCTION

You may feel you want a quick remedy for your bulges and decide to seek medical help via the private sector. A private doctor, who is likely to be more sympathetic towards the problem than your GP, may recommend plastic surgery. This can work to a certain extent, but before you take drastic action and resort to the knife (or, in the case of liposuction, the 'suction tube'), you must convince yourself that nothing else works for you. Liposuction, like any operation, can be uncomfortable, even painful, initially. You may also need to take a good look at your bank balance as private medicine doesn't come cheap.

You must ensure that the surgeon of your choice is reputable. We hear many stories through the news media of plastic surgery having disastrous results. One of the ways of finding a good surgeon is on your own GP's recommendation, but you may have to battle with him or her to get one as many GPs are opposed to cosmetic surgery in any shape or form. If your doctor won't recommend anyone, you may be interested in a booklet recently published called *The Independent Guide to Cosmetic Surgery* by Joanna Gibbon. This gives a list of fully qualified plastic surgeons, all of whom are members of the British Association of Aesthetic Plastic Surgeons. I would strongly recommend that you choose a surgeon from this list rather than going via an advertisement in a glossy magazine – good surgeons don't need to advertise!

Don't ever go to a surgeon 'cold'. You must never be afraid to ask to see samples of their handiwork in the form of photographs. You have to know that what you will have done on your own body will give you pleasure and not an unsightly scar which will last for life and depress you every time you look at it. In liposuction, the scar is generally ½" (0.5 cm–1 cm) in length and should not really be noticeable.

A good surgeon will discuss the operation with you and will tell you if your skin type is unsuitable for certain cosmetic surgery. You should never be pressurized and you should be given time to think over the pros and cons. If you can, visit a few surgeons. Don't rush into cosmetic surgery half-heartedly and as prices for liposuction vary, do shop around, but you can reckon on spending approximately £1,600.

You must also remember that the younger your skin, the better the results will be. You need to have good elasticity – but again, the surgeon of your choice should discuss this with you.

The operation itself is relatively quick, but of course this depends on the amount of fat to be 'sucked' out. It may involve an overnight stay in hospital. About half an hour before the operation, you will be given a 'pre-med' injection to calm you. The operation is usually carried out under a general anaesthetic. A small cut or cuts will be made, depending on the amount to be drained, and a tube inserted. Fat is then taken from the affected area(s). During the operation, you will be put into a specially designed girdle to prevent possible 'sagging'. This usually stays in place for approximately three weeks. Initially you will experience a certain amount of discomfort, but as the days wear on, the pain wears off. You can reckon on being 'out of action' for approximately two weeks.

If you choose well and your skin is suitable, the results can be superb; however the cellulite/fat may return if you again put on too much weight.

ABDOMINOPLASTY

If your problem area is around your middle an abdominoplasty or 'tummy tuck' can be performed. This again is a drastic measure and should only be considered when all else fails. Perhaps the skin around the abdomen has been stretched out of all proportion during pregnancy, or the body was once much heavier and rapid weight loss has caused the skin to droop and sag. If you have toned up your abdominal muscles but the skin still hangs, only then perhaps should you consider plastic surgery. If this is the case, and if you are in your late thirties or older, you may be an ideal candidate.

This is not a pleasant operation and you will be required to stay in hospital for two or three days. After that, you will be incapacitated for approximately three to four weeks. An incision is made from the hip to the public bone and up towards the other hip. In almost all cases the muscles are tightened up as well as the skin. If too much excess skin has to be removed, the navel may have to be repositioned. Again, a specially designed girdle is worn for twelve to fourteen days after the operation to keep the skin taut. In a few rare cases the patient may have to undergo another minor operation at a later date to revise the scar around the navel or to correct 'dog ears' on scar corners around the abdomen.

The cost of an abdominoplasty is in the region of £2,500.

SAUNA SUITS? NO!

Sauna suits can seriously damage your health, and my only reason for mentioning them here is to urge you to have nothing to do with them!

You may read advertisements for sauna suits offering rash promises that they will help you lose weight. This is a fallacy: all they will help you lose is money. They are dangerous and should not, in any circumstances, be used.

Some fitness trainers I have come across encourage their students to work in these death traps and then tell them to go and sit in a sauna. I can't express strongly enough just how dangerous they are – *don't buy them*. If your trainer tells you to wear one, get rid of him or her. No trainer who recommends them knows what they're talking about! Sauna suits will make you lose water only, not fat; as soon as you take a drink, the lost fluid returns!

There have been fatalities through people wearing sauna suits. The body perspires in order to take the body temperature down; sweat on the skin's surface will do this. If perspiration is trapped between your skin and a 'sauna suit', it can't escape and your body overheats, with obvious disastrous results.

Heat-induced illness can cause widespread irreversible tissue damage in the body. This was brought to light in an unfortunate incident during an army training exercise in England in 1986. Trainee divers were put through a 20-minute exercise regime wearing pants, vest and boots. They then changed into standard Royal Navy dry diving suits worn over woollen jumpsuits and were asked to run across mud-flats. The course was 0.8 mile, which they were expected to complete in 15 minutes. Before the finish, one of the men – a 17-year-old – collapsed with breathing problems, another two followed suit. The 17-year-old died from the effects of excessive heat; the other two recovered after hospital treatment. Obviously we wouldn't wear woollens underneath a sauna suit, but the prinicple remains the same.

'Heat illness may rapidly progress to a disastrous situation with widespread tissue damage and sudden death without correct and prompt treatment.' (This quotation is taken from 'Exertional Hyperpyrexia: Case Report and Review of Pathophysiological Mechanisms', by M.R. Jarmulowicz and J.D. Buchanan; Surgeon Lieutenant Jarmulowicz is on the Emergency List: Surgeon Commander Buchanan is Consultant Adviser in Pathology to MDG(N) and is serving at RNH Haslar). Sauna suits work in exactly the same way as diving suits. The heat cannot dissipate and so the body overheats with disastrous, sometimes fatal, results. You should *never* wear them; you won't lose weight, you will lose water, and this is instantly replaced when you take a drink. Don't waste your money – you can never 'spot' reduce, and you may just not live to regret it!

I've seen women in the Turkish baths near where I live sitting in sauna suits or swathed in black bin-liners frantically trying to lose weight. When I've told them of the dangers, they won't believe me and remain determined to sweat off their fat no matter what. There really should be a health warning pasted up; 'sauna suits can seriously damage your health'. Perhaps when someone reads this section there will be!

If you need any more evidence, let me refer you to research carried out in the United States on 'vapour barrier coveralls': 'The quality of impermeability to vapor puts the user of these garments at risk for heat stress because the vapor barrier effectively prevents sweat evaporation and thus limits the most important heat dissipation mechanisms under conditions of heavy muscular work in a warm environment. In addition, like other garments, they may increase risk for heat stress by preventing convective heat lost'. (This quotation is taken from 'Heat Stress Association with the use of Vapor-Barrier Garments', by William S. Beckett MD, John E. Davis PhD, Neil Vroman PhD, Robert Nadig MD and Suzanne Fortney PhD.)

Also, don't think you can lose weight by endlessly sitting in a sauna. 'Spending too long in the hot room is dangerous, and one young man developed renal failure after spending five hours in the sauna in a futile attempt to lose weight' quoted Clifford Hawkins in the British Medical *Journal* Volume 295, (24th October 1987).

APPENDIX:
FOOD AND DRUGS

If you've read right through this book you should be in no doubt by now of the huge importance to your size, your health and your general well-being of what you eat and drink. I didn't weigh you down with too much detail in the earlier chapters as I wanted you to grasp the essentials and then get to grips with the programme and get on your way to results. However, it is worth knowing more about what you put into your body – not only in terms of food and drink, but also in the form of drugs – both those we think of as drugs and those we take for granted as everyday substances. So read on and find out what you're really putting into your mouth!

FATS
What are fats? Basically they are the most concentrated source of energy supplied to the body.

Fats make foods more palatable. A dry scone alone can be pretty boring, but spread it with butter and jam and add to this a dollop of double Devon cream and it becomes much more interesting and is much easier to eat. However, it also becomes lethal: who can stop at one? Cream teas are very 'moreish'. The more you eat, the more you want. You taste the fat in the cream and the sweetness of the jam and keep going until all of a sudden you realize you've eaten too much, too late! You wish you'd never started. You feel bloated and uncomfortable, so what do you do? Try to get rid of it through exercise? You must be joking, you sit down and wallow and hope the feeling of resemblance to a beached whale will soon disappear. However, the more you sit and wallow after a binge, the worse you'll become. The excess fat and carbohydrates settle on you as great blobs of excess fat. And they're not fussy where they settle. If you add a few glasses of alcohol to revive you after your binge, you'll help the spare tyre along nicely – you'll expand in all directions (the calorie content in alcohol is extremely high).

So what do we do? Can we find an ideal diet that we can eat, but be happy that our waists will never expand? Unfortunately not. No diet will 'spot' reduce. You can't take in certain food with the instruction 'don't settle on the bum or tum'. If your food intake is more than your body actually needs to function, this will be stored in a reserve or storehouse for an emergency – when you need a sudden burst of energy. However, there are a lot of overstocked 'storehouses' which, generally speaking, will never be called upon to be used. The more we eat and the less exercise we take, the more lethargic and sluggish we become.

Fat stores itself willy nilly in all your nooks and crannies: sometimes on your legs, sometimes on your bottom and more often than not around your middle. There are, however, 'sensible eating' diets which offer extremely good results. If you watch your intake of fats, sugars, salts and carbohydrates and have a good balance of fresh fruit and vegetables, you are well on the way to a good, safe eating pattern and one which will have lasting results. If however, you load up on full-fat dairy produce, you'll have more than your fair share of physiological problems.

There is a lot of controversy concerning the respective values of animal fats and vegetables fats, and it's easy to become confused when we read media reports of what is best for us and try to separate the marketing ploys from the facts. So what are the differences?

Basically, there are three types of fat:

1. Saturated fats, obtained from animal produce. These increase the amount of cholesterol in the body, which in turn will lead to heart-related problems.
2. Polyunsaturated fats, obtained from fish and vegetables and usually found in liquid form when stored at room temperature. This type of fat helps lower blood fat levels. The 1984 Committee on the Medical Aspects of Food (COMA) recommends we increase our intake of polyunsaturates from 5 per cent to 7 per cent.
3. Monounsaturated fats, also usually in liquid form at room temperature, though they may solidify if put in a cold place. Found in high levels in avocados and olive oil. Recent studies show that they may help lower blood fat levels.

It is the saturated fats that you should avoid, as these are the ones that encourage the build-up of high cholesterol levels, which in turn contribute towards heart disease.

As a guide, the table shows the percentage of fatty acids present in different animal fats and vegetable oils.

	Saturated	*Polyunsaturated*	*Monounsaturated*
Vegetable oils:			
Corn oil	15	60	25
Maize oil	14	59	28
Olive oil	15	10	75

	Saturated	Polyunsaturated	Monounsaturated
Palm oil	47	9	44
Peanut oil	18	30	48
Saffflower oil	9	78	13
Sesame oil	16	43	41
Soya oil	15	52	25
Sunflower oil	11	72	16
Animal fats:			
Butter	60	3	32
Beef fat	45	4	50
Chicken fat	35	15	48
Duck fat	29	13	57
Herring oil	22	20	56
Lamb fat	52	5	41
Lard	40	9	44
Mackerel oil	27	29	41
Pork fat	42	8	48
Turkey fat	36	34	27

CHOLESTEROL

We make approximately 80 per cent of cholesterol in our own livers, and while you can lower your cholesterol level by taking in less fatty food, to reduce it appreciably you do in fact have to make fairly drastic changes affecting your whole lifestyle, including reducing stressful situations and taking a lot more exercise. Exercise can in fact help reduce stress by getting rid of your frustrations in a positive way and achieving good physical changes. Lowering your fat intake alone will make only a minimal difference if your lifestyle remains the same. However, it's a start if you do have a high cholesterol count. And if you do happen to have any form of heart-related illness in your family and are over forty it's a good idea to have your cholesterol level measured. It seems you could also do worse than eat more carrots: 'The latest information to support carrots is the news that they contain calcium pectate, a type of fibre which helps reduce cholesterol levels. Calcium pectate is also found in onions, broccoli and cabbage. American researchers (why do they always seem to be American?) say that eating two carrots a day can reduce cholesterol levels by 10 to 20 per cent. Carrots are a versatile vegetable and can be served raw, whole or grated in salads, or cooked and used in stir fry dishes and pizza toppings. As with all vegetables the less they are cooked, the better they are nutritionally' (*Health & Fitness* magazine, February 1990).

Eating fatty fish such as kippers, mackerel, salmon and herrings can play an important role in preventing fatal heart attacks. 'A modest intake of fatty fish – two or three portions per week – may reduce mortality in men who have recovered from a heart attack', *The Lancet*'s researchers have discovered. This is because Omega-3, the name given to essential fatty acids, are polyunsaturated acids which can actually help to break down our cholesterol level. Auriel Mott explains:

The Omega-3 fatty acids in fish are called

> eicosapentaenoic acid (EPA)
> docosapentaenoic acid (DPA)
> and   docosahexaenoic acid (DHA).

How Omega-3 fatty acids work to reduce the risk of heart disease is as follows. To begin with, they act on the body's cholesterol levels. Cholesterol is made by the liver as well as being absorbed from fatty foods in the diet. But not all cholesterol is bad for you. There are two main types of cholesterol – low density lipoproteins (LDLs), which are harmful because they clog the arteries, and high-density lipoproteins (HDLs) which are helpful because they encourage the liver to eliminate LDLs, thereby preventing the clogging process. EPA has been found to lower LDLs and to raise the beneficial HDLs.

In addition, the EPA 'thins' the blood by reducing the stickiness of the platelets in the blood. These platelets are part of the blood clotting process in the body.

DPA also appears to have a relaxing effect on the smooth muscle of the blood vessels, which may explain why fish oils seem to have a favourable effect on those people suffering from moderate hypertension. (*Vitamin Connection*, January/February 1990)

Get into the habit of checking food labels to see how high or low oils and fats come on the list of ingredients – (NB low-fat spreads are *not* high in polyunsaturated fat! They are lower in fat because they are 50 per cent water. As prices are similar, you are better off simply using less of the original!)

A good rule of thumb is to try to reduce as far as possible the intake of all dairy and animal fat produce: cheese, full fat milk, fatty meat, cream, butter. *Fat is stored as fat!*

The following information, supplied by dietitians at Safeway plc, shows you how to substitute lower-fat alternatives into your diet:

High fat food	*Lower-fat alternatives*
Cream, double	Low-fat yogurt
Cheddar cheese	Cottage cheese
Chocolate cake	Bread
Potatoes, chipped	Potatoes, baked in skins

High fat food	Lower-fat alternatives
Potato crisps	Apple
Milk chocolate	Orange
Beef steak, fried	Beef steak, stewed
Haddock, fried	Haddock, steamed
Bacon, streaky, fried	Chicken, roast (minus skin)
Egg yolk	Egg white
Milk, whole	Milk, skimmed or semi- skimmed.

If you find it difficult to switch to low-fat alternatives, reduce drastically the amount of animal fat you use. Spread butter thinly – literally scrape it over your toast – and slice cheese paper-thin. Try to make the change-overs in your own time otherwise you'll hate what you eat. You have to enjoy what goes into your mouth. It's no use eating endless salads because you've read they're good for you and becoming miserable because you crave for a 'Desperate Dan'-type cow pie. Become more aware and make the changes gradually. The important thing is knowing what is good and bad for your body and doing something about changing your whole lifestyle.

SALT

Take a look at the day's intake shown in the following table and note the salt content, remembering that all we need is 1 g of salt per day as recommended by the Health Education Authority!

	Salt, g
Breakfast	
2 slices toast and butter, tea	0.9
Mid-morning coffee and 2 biscuits	0.2
1 packet crisps	0.5
Lunch	
Chicken soup (1 pint packet)	3.0
2 slices bread and butter	0.9
Afternoon	
2 biscuits and tea	0.2
Supper	
Steak and kidney pie	2.3
Canned sweet corn	0.6
Canned peas	0.4
2 glasses wine	
Bedtime	
Milky drink and 2 biscuits	0.2
TOTAL	9.2

Add to that the salt content in sauces, mustard and chutneys and you can see how most people's daily intake goes way over our recommended 1 g. Five grams is the equivalent to one fifth of a teaspoon; the average person's daily intake is somewhere in the region of just over two to three teaspoonsful.

If you take in this amount of salt, and especially if you're a smoker and your family history shows heart-related illnesses, you could be an ideal candidate for heart problems!

Your diet can easily be altered to reduce salt intake by making a few radical changes. Avoid eating tinned and prepared products. These are usually loaded with salt and fat. Cut out or drastically reduce snacks and biscuits, which also cling to your teeth long after they've been eaten – more so even than chocolate. Instead, get into the habit of including cereals, pulses, fresh fruit and raw vegetables into your diet: make your intestines work. Keep a supply of crudités (prepared raw vegetables) or your favourite fruits in the fridge. Experiment with exotic fruits if you're bored with the run-of-the-mill ones. If you pay over the odds for them, I'm sure they will be eaten! If you find you absolutely crave for one of your treats, buy it, cut it into pieces and limit yourself to one small piece a day – make it last, rather than devouring the whole lot in one go.

Little cutbacks here and there will definitely help ring the changes. If you take something away completely, you'll crave it all the more. If you have a little, you can make it last. (Very similar to a good love affair: always hold something back!)

The following is a brief guide that can be used as a checklist when you go shopping. Try to avoid high-sodium foods, go carefully on the medium-sodium food and try to choose more from the low-sodium section. Note that butter is 2% salt; and vegetables have a lower salt content than meat.

High sodium foods
Smoked meat – bacon, sausages, corned beef, ham, salami
Tinned or smoked fish
Bread (obviously, brands differ)
Butter, margarine and low-fat spread (unless marked 'unsalted')
Hard cheese
Some breakfast cereal e.g. cornflakes, All-Bran, Rice Krispies
Savoury biscuits
Self-raising flour
Bicarbonate of soda
Olives
Tomato ketchup
Prepared mustard
Stock cubes (highest ingredient is usually salt)

Medium-sodium foods
Eggs
Fresh meat
Fresh fish
Celery, carrots, beetroot, turnips, watercress
Cottage cheese
Cream cheese
Milk
Wine and beer (when drunk in large quantities; one glass is OK)
Dried fruit, unsoaked (in large amounts)
Canned vegetables
Mayonnaise

Low-sodium foods
All vegetables (except olives and those listed under medium-sodium
    foods)
Cooked beans (uncanned)
Cooked dried fruit
All fresh fruit
Wheat, rice and other cereals
Shredded Wheat, Puffed Wheat, porridge, muesli
Nuts (unsalted)
Cream

CARBOHYDRATES

Carbohydrates – starches and sugars – are eaten to provide our bodies with energy. When we 'overload' and don't use up what isn't needed in the form of exercise, we store the excess as fat in the fatty layer of our bodies. Carbohydrates teamed up with fats provide the source of most of the surplus calories and consequently surplus fat cells.

The following table gives a brief summary of information from a book produced by the British Diabetic Association called *Countdown*. It gives the amount of carbohydrates in grams and also the number of calories present in some common food and drink items.

Item	Quantity	Carbohydrates	Calories
BISCUITS			
Allinson Carob Fruit & Nut	1	9	85
Appleford's Peanut/Almond Cluster bar	1	15	140
Bahlsen Choco Leibniz, plain	1	9	72
Bejam Custard Creams	1	9	60
Boots Digestive Creams	1	9	62
Burton's Coconut Delights	1	16	105
Cadbury's Orange Creams	1	10	80
Crawford's Bourbon Creams	1	10	63
Jacob's 'Club' Milk	1	15	117
Marks & Spencer Break In	1	14	119
McVitie United Extra Time	1	29	223
Nabisco Happy Faces	1	11	77
Peek Freans Custard Creams	1	16	53
Quaker Harvest Chewy Bars with apple & raisin	1	17	110
Safeway Orange Sandwich	1	17	130
Sainsbury Thistle Shortbread	1	12	105
Tesco Flapjack	1	20	135
Waitrose Wafer Sandwich with chocolate filling	1	13	85
Walker's Highland Shortbread	1	15	118
CONFECTIONERY			
Dolly Mixtures	1 oz	25	110
Jelly Babies	1 oz	25	95
Jelly Beans	1 oz	25	105
Allinson Carob Crunch Bar	1	22	150
Bassett's Liquorice Allsorts	113 g	90	390
Bassett's Wine Gums	4 oz	90	370
Boots Barley Sugar Drops	1	5	20
Boots Glucose Drops	1	6	22
Boots Milk Choc Bar with Fruit Muesli	1 bar	34	170
Cadbury's Caramel	50 g bar	32	245
Cadbury's Crunchie (standard)	1 bar	26	165
Cadbury's Milk Fruit & Nut	100 g bar	57	470
Dextrosol, all flavours	1	3	12

Item	Quantity	Carbohydrates	Calories
Fox's Glacier Mints (from 113 g pack)	1	5	20
Granose Carob Fruit Bar	35 g bar	26	145
Littlewoods Fudge	35 g bar	25	140
Marks & Spencer Liqueur Truffles	200 g pack	85	1040
M&S Milk Chocolate Buttons	75 g bag	45	385
M&S Popcorn	35 g bag	30	120
M&S Walnut Whip	1	15	130
Mars Bar (standard)	1 bar	48	310
Galaxy	50 g bar	28	275
Topic	1 bar	32	265
Nestle's Milky Bar	1 oz bar	16	155
Kit Kat	large bar	31	250
Munchies	1 pkt	3	25
Smarties	small tube	26	160
Walnut Whip, milk	1	22	170
Safeway Chocolate Brazils, milk	1	4	55
Safeway Chocolate Brazils, plain	1	5	55
Sainsbury's Devon Toffees	8 oz	160	1040
Sharps Extra Strong Mints	1	3	10
Wrigley's Spearmint Gum	1 stk	2	10
Trebor Cough Candy Twist	1	7	26
Trebor Mints	1	1	6

SOFT DRINKS
(fizzy, sweetened)

Item	Quantity	Carbohydrates	Calories
Lemonade	½ pt	19	70
Indian Tonic Water	½ pt	18	65
Bitter Lemon	½ pt	25	100
Ginger Beer	½ pt	22	85
Shandy	½ pt	15	75
Britvic Orange	300 ml	39	145
Coca Cola	330 ml	35	135
Lilt	330 ml	38	155
Corona Coola	330 ml	38	140
Littlewoods Tizer	330 ml	34	130
Marks & Spencer Sparkling Orange Drink	320 ml	48	190
Pepsi Cola	330 ml	37	145

Item	Quantity	Carbohydrates	Calories
Schweppes Sparking Orange Crush	330 ml	39	150
Tango Sparkling Orange	330 ml	40	155
Top Deck Lemonade & Cider	330 ml	28	125
FRUIT JUICES			
Britvic Pineapple Juice	250 ml	35	130
Coca Cola Five Alive Citrus	1 ltr	125	480
Heinz Grapefruit Juice, sweetened	120 ml	20	80
Kellogg's Rise & Shine	60 g sachet	53	200
Libby's Orange 'C', sweetened	930 ml	125	475
Schweppes Tomato juice cocktail	180 ml	8	30
ICE CREAM			
1 scoop minimum	10	80	
1 scoop maximum	15	120	
Birds Eye Arctic Circles	1	21	155
Lyons Maid Gold Seal chocolate swirl	1 pot	185	1170
King Cone, chocolate	1	26	220
Safeway Cornish cutting brick	1 portion	9	70
Tesco Choc Ice	1	13	130
Waitrose Sorbet, blackcurrant	1	16	70
Walls Cornetto, mint choc chip	1	24	225
CAKES			
Cadbury's Chocolate Whirls	1	18	130
Cadbury's Mini Rolls	1	16	115
Littlewoods Cherry Bakewell	1	31	200
Lyons Jam Tart	1	25	140
M&S Chorley Cakes	1	40	290
M&S Egg Custard Tart	1	27	230
M&S Mini Rum Babas	1	47	250
Mr Kipling Battenburg Treats	1	30	175
Safeway Trifle Sponge	1	18	80
Tesco Angel Layer Cake	1 oz	16	115
Vitbe Raisin Brans	1	23	155
DESSERTS			
Ambrosia Chocolate Desserts	1 pot	21	140

Item	Quantity	Carbohydrates	Calories
Ambrosia Creamed Rice	170 g tin	30	155
Bejam Knickerbocker Glory	1	45	275
Birds Trifle Mix	1 pkt	125	620
Brown & Polson Instant Custard Mix	90 g sachet	80	420
Chambourcy Chocolate Cream Dessert	1 pot	23	140
Eden Vale Blackcurrant Cheesecake	100 g	25	220
Heinz Chocolate Sponge Pudding	300 g	135	890
HP Chocolate Dessert	1 tbsp	11	45
M&S Creme Caramel	1 pot	27	190
Robertsons Christmas Pudding	227 g	120	675
Ross Apple Dumplings	1	50	335

SNACKS AND NUTS

Item	Quantity	Carbohydrates	Calories
Booker Health Barbara's Cookies, Oatmeal & Raisin	1	23	228
Golden Wonder Crisps, all flavours	25 g pkt	10	125
Jacket crisps, all flavours	1 pkt	12	155
Wotsits, all flavours	1 pkt	15	130
Holland & Barrett Bombay Mix	1 oz	8	140
Desert Island Delight	1 oz	9	160
Holly Mill Muesli square snack	1	32	220
Jordans Original Crunchy Bars, with orange and carob	1	17	140
KP Dry Roasted Peanuts	50 g pkt	5	280
Hula Hoops, all flavours	30 g pkt	18	160
Mixed nuts and raisins	50 g pkt	11	245
Littlewoods Burger bites	50 g pkt	30	275
Pizza Bites	50 g pkt	30	275
Marks & Spencer Californian Corn Chips	75 g pkt	40	420
Pistachio nuts	60 g pkt	12	360
Prawn Cocktail Snacks	50 g pkt	25	245
McVitie's Mini Cheddars	30 g pkt	16	160
Phileas Fogg Californian Corn Chips	40 g pkt	20	225
Safeway Savoury Puffs	50 g pkt	20	300

Item	Quantity	Carbohydrates	Calories
Sainsbury Potato Squares	50 g pkt	30	275
Ready salted potato chips	75 g pkt	42	390
Smiths Crisps, all flavours	1 pkt	12	150
Cheezers	1 pkt	12	150
Monster Munch, all flavours	1 pkt	17	155
Tesco Bacon Bites	50 g pkt	35	225
Onion Rings	50 g pkt	32	250
Waitrose Cheese Puffs	50 g pkt	25	300
Walkers Crisps, all flavours	28 g pkt	15	160
PASTRY GOODS (one portion)			
Birds Eye Chicken Pie	1	33	410
Bowyers Chicken and Ham Pie	1	40	415
Bowyers Meat & Vegetable Pie	1	50	575
Bowyers Pork Pie	140 g	38	640
Bowyers Sausage Roll (individual)	1	17	275
Kraft Ploughman's Pasty	1	35	440
Marks & Spencer Minced Beef Pie	1 small	32	575
M&S Quiche Lorraine	1 indiv.	26	495
Ross Cornish Pasty	1	20	240
Safeway Steak & Kidney Pudding	1 small	40	430
Tesco Meat & Potato Pie	145 g	38	435
Waitrose Chicken, Ham and Mushroom Pie	5 oz	30	335
SAUCES (level teaspoon and tablespoon)			
Apple sauce	tbsp	3	10
Brown sauce	tbsp	5	20
Cranberry sauce	tsp	2	10
Creamed horseradish sauce	tsp	1	10
Fruity sauce	tbsp	5	20
Horseradish sauce	tsp	neg	5
Mayonnaise	tbsp	neg	100
Mint jelly	tsp	5	15
Mint sauce	tsp	neg	5
Redcurrant jelly	tsp	4	15
Salad cream	tbsp	3	50
Tartare sauce	tbsp	3	40
Tomato ketchup	tbsp	5	20

Item	Quantity	Carbohydrates	Calories
YOGURTS			
Chambourcy (Nouvelle)			
black cherry	150 g pot	24	120
Chambourcy peach & redcurrant	150 g pot	28	140
Eden Vale Gold Ski, all flavours	150 g pot	28	180
Eden Vale Munch Bunch apple	125 g pot	33	155
Fage Total Greek Yogurt:			
Sheep's milk	225 g tub	9	210
Strained cow's milk	225 g tub	9	305
Loseley Low Fat hazelnut	150 g pot	21	130
Marks & Spencer Low Fat			
raspberry ripple	150 g pot	32	190
M&S Thick & Creamy, all flavours	150 g pot	29	160
Safeway Low Fat tropical fruit	150 g pot	30	150
Sainsbury Low Fat rhubarb	150 g pot	27	145
St Ivel Real, all flavours	125 g pot	17	105
Tesco Low Fat pineapple	150 g pot	22	125
Tesco Real French set yogurt	125 g pot	16	100
Waitrose Creamy Yogurt,			
all flavours	125 g pot	25	175–185
Yoplait Breakfast Yogurt,			
all flavours	140 g pot	23	145
Yop Drinking Yogurt	200 ml	25	165
CEREALS			
Kellogg's Cornflakes	1 oz	24	100
Birds Grape Nuts	1 oz	22	100
Force Wheatflakes	1 oz	24	110
Granose Crunchy Nut Cereal	1 oz	17	140
Kellogg's All Bran	1 oz	13	70
Lyons Tetley Ready Brek Original	1 oz	21	110
Nabisco Shredded Wheat	1	16	80
Prewett's Bran Muesli	1 oz	16	95
Shreddies	1 oz	21	95
Quaker Puffed Wheat	1 oz	20	95
Safeway Rice Crunchies	1 oz	24	100
Sainsbury Rice Pops	1 oz	23	100

SUGAR

Sugar is a source of energy: but of nothing else! Taken in excess it turns into, and is stored as, fat. Sugar is classed as 'empty calorie' food. It has no nutritional value and can upset the appetite. There is no fibre in a chocolate bar and therefore it won't make you feel full; sick yes, but full no! If you crave chocolates or biscuits, eat them at the end of a meal rather than picking between meals – one, two then perhaps the whole box! with luck you'll soon rid yourself of the habit!

If you keep chocolate, keep it in the fridge and limit yourself to a small slice off a bar or a couple of squares off a block. Don't eat the whole lot. Make one bar or block last the week. Get your willpower in working order! If you know your 'treat' has to be stretched out, you'll persevere.

The following table gives you a rough idea of the hidden sugar in what you eat and drink. (This information is taken from McCance & Widdowson *The Composition of Foods* (4th revised edition), edited by A.A. Paul and D.A.T. Southgate; *Carbohydrate Countdown 1977*, published by the British Diabetic Association; and manufacturers' information. The figures are meant as a rough guide only and were correct at the time of going to press.)

Product	Quantity	Sugar content, in teaspoons
BISCUITS (per biscuit)		
Chocolate Digestive	1	1¾
Chocolate Wheatmeal	1 small	1
Digestive	1	½
Ginger Nut	1	1
Jaffa Cake	1	1½
Lincoln	1	½
Rich Tea	1	½
Shortcake	1	½
Chocolate Wafer	1	¾
Cream Cracker	1	trace
Hovis	1	1/10
Ritz	5	¼
CONFECTIONERY		
Aero	1 bar	3½
Banjo	2 biscuits	2¾
Boiled sweets	1 tube	10
Bounty	2 pieces	3¾
Caramel	1 bar (50 g)	5½
Chocolate, milk	1 bar (38 g)	3½

Product	Quantity	Sugar content, in teaspoons
Chocolate, fruit & nut	1 bar (50 g)	4
Chocolate, whole nut	1 bar (50 g)	4
Chocolate, plain	1 bar (50 g)	6
Chocolate Cream	1 bar (45 g)	7
Crunchie	1 bar (40 g)	6
Dolly Mixtures	1 box (113 g)	20½
Double Decker	1 bar (48 g)	6
Drifter	1 pkt (45 g)	6½
Fruit Gums	1 tube (35 g)	3
Fruit Pastilles	1 tube (40 g)	6¼
Galaxy	1 bar (50 g)	3¾
Kit Kat	1 bar (45 g)	3¾
Liquorice Allsorts	1 box (113 g)	17¾
Lion Bar	1 bar (45 g)	5½
Maltesers	1 pkt (40 g)	2½
Mars Bar	1 bar (59 g)	5
Milky Way	1 bar (28 g)	1½
Murray Mints	1 pkt (50 g)	10
Picnic	1 bar (45 g)	4¾
Polo Mints	1 tube (25 g)	5
Polo	1 tube (46 g)	5½
Slush Puppie	1 sm cup (207 ml)	6¼
Smarties	1 tube (35 g)	4¼
Snickers	1 bar (46 g)	3½
Star Bar	1 bar (45 g)	4½
Ticket	1 bar (53 g)	6
Topic	1 bar (48 g)	3¾
Treets	1 pkt (45 g)	4½
Twix	1 pkt (45 g)	3½
Turkish Delight	1 bar (52 g)	7¾
Yorkie	1 bar (60 g)	5¾
SOFT DRINKS		
Apeel Orange Drink	1 pkt (100 g)	16¾
Apeel Orange Drink	1 glass (10 g)	1¾
Blackcurrant Cordial	1 glass (40 g)	5
Bitter Lemon	1 bottle (240 g)	5¾
Coca Cola	1 can (330 g)	7
Strike Cola	1½ glass (330 g)	5½
Ginger Ale	1 bottle (240 g)	4¼

Product	Quantity	Sugar content, in teaspoons
Ginger Beer	1 can (330 g)	7
Lemonade	1 glass (220 g)	3¼
Lemon Squash	1 glass (40 g)	2¼
Orange Squash	1 glass (40 g)	2½
Lucozade	1 glass (200 g)	7¾
Ribena	1 glass (40 g)	5
Tizer	1 glass (200 g)	4¼
Tonic Water	1 bottle (240 g)	4
Vimto	1 glass (200 g)	2¾
Milk Shakes	1 pkt (40 g)	3¾
Milk Shakes	½ pt made up (20 g)	2
SPREADS		
Chocolate spread	2 tsp	2¼
Honey	2 tsp	2¼
Jam	2 tsp	2
Lemon curd	2 tsp	2
Marmalade	2 tsp	2¼
Peanut butter	3 tsp	¼
Syrup	2 tsp	2½
Treacle	2 tsp	2½
BREAKFAST CEREALS		
All Bran	1 oz	1
Branflakes	6 tbsp	¾
Cornflakes	6 tbsp	¼
Muesli	2 tbsp	1½
Puffed Wheat	6 tbsp	trace
Rice Krispies	6 tbsp	¼
Shredded Wheat	1 biscuit	trace
Shreddies	2 tbsp	½
Special K	6 tbsp	¼
Sugar Puffs	6 tbsp	2¼
Weetabix	1 biscuit	trace
CAKES		
Sponge cake	1 med. slice	1½
Scone	1	½
Sandwich cake	1 med. slice	4½
Lemon meringue pie	1 med. slice	3¼
Currant bun	1	1¼
Chocolate cake	1 med. slice	1¾

Product	Quantity	Sugar content, in teaspoons
DESSERTS		
Angel Delight	1 pkt	7¾
Chocolate sauce	3 tsp	2
Dream Topping	1 sachet	1¾
Ice cream	300 g	9
Strawberry Sauce	3 tsp	1¼
Instant custard	1 pkt	6¾
Instant Whip	1 pkt	10½
Jelly	1 pkt	18¾
Tinned fruit	213 g	5
Trifle mix	40 g	3½
Fruit Yogurt	150 g	4½
Fruit-flavoured yoghurt	150 g	2¾
Tinned rice pudding	220 g	2½
BEVERAGES		
Bournvita	3 tsp	1½
Drinking Chocolate	3 tsp	2½
Horlicks	3 tsp	1
Ovaltine	3 tsp	1
Coffee & Chicory Essence	3 tsp	1
SAUCES, PICKLES, ETC.		
Brown Sauce	3 tsp	¾
Fruity Sauce	3 tsp	¾
Salad Cream	3 tsp	½
Sweet Pickle	3 tsp	¾
Sweet Piccallili	3 tsp	½
Sweet Military Pickle	3 tsp	1
Pickled Walnuts	3 tsp	¼
Tomato Ketchup	3 tsp	¾
Worcestershire Sauce	3 tsp	¼
SOUPS		
Tinned chicken soup	200 g	½
Tinned tomato soup	200 g	1
Tinned vegetable soup	200 g	1
Packet chicken soup	20 g	½
Packet Minestrone	15 g	½
Packet Oxtail	15 g	1½
Packet Tomato	20 g	2

Product	Quantity	Sugar content, in teaspoons
TINNED VEGETABLES		
Baked beans	225 g	2
Butter beans	213 g	trace
Kidney beans	213 g	1½
Peas	213 g	½
Sweet corn	100 g	1½
TINNED MEAT		
Corned beef	340 g	¾
STOCK CUBES		
Chicken	1 cube	trace
Beef	1 cube	trace

VITAMINS AND MINERALS

It is said that the British and Americans have the most expensive urine in the world as a result of our intake of added vitamins and minerals in the form of pills. If we take in supplements when they are not required by the body, we pee them away. Of course, during pregnancy and old age and with certain medical conditions these are usually recommended, but the majority of us don't need them.

VITAMINS AND MINERALS IN PACKAGED FOODS

The information which follows was provided by Safeway Food Stores Ltd in their guide on 'Nutritional Labelling'.

When applicable, vitamin and mineral contents will also be included in the nutritional information panel. They will appear in the format shown below. This example shows wholemeal bread:

NUTRITIONAL INFORMATION

Average values	Per 100g	Per slice
Energy	882 kj (210 kcal)	261 kj (62 kcal)
Protein	9.5 g	2.8 g
Carbohydrate	45.6 g	13.5 g
Fibre	8.5 g	2.5 g
Fat	2.6 g	0.8 g
Thiamin	25%	
Niacin	29%	
Iron	36%	
Calcium	21%	

The Recommended Daily Amount (RDA) of vitamins and minerals is the amount of vitamin or mineral which should be consumed daily by an average adult man to prevent any type of deficiency developing and to ensure good health. The values are determined by the Department of Health and Social Security (DHSS) and printed in the Government labelling regulations. They are only provided for those nutrients for which a minimum average requirement has been determined and the RDA is generally about 10 per cent above this minimum to allow for individual variation.

The vitamins which may be claimed in the nutrition sections of our labels are:

	RDA *(for the average adult)*
Vitamin A (Retinol)	750.0 mg
Thiamin (Vitamin B1)	1.2 mg
Riboflavin (Vitamin B2)	1.6 mg
Niacin (Nicotinic acid)	18.0 mg
Folic acid	300.0 mg
Vitamin B12	2.0 mg
Vitamin C (Ascorbic acid)	30.0 mg
Vitamin D (Cholecalciferol)	2.5 mg

The minerals which may be claimed are:

Calcium	500.0 mg
Iodine	140.0 mg
Iron	12.0 mg

Generally we only make a claim when the stated serving will provide at least one sixth or 17 per cent of the daily requirement for that vitamin or mineral.

1 mg (milligram) = 1/1000 g; 1 mg (microgram) = 1/1000 mg.

WHERE TO GET YOUR VITAMINS

Vitamin A
Liver, dark green leafy vegetables (including dandelion leaves which are a mild diuretic), carrots, yellow fruit, margarine, cooked spinach, fatty fish, full-fat milk and cheeses made from it. Vitamin A can be toxic if taken in excess.

Vitamin C
Citrus fruit: oranges, lemons, grapefruit; blackcurrants, strawberries,

tomatoes, potatoes, leafy green vegetables, red and green peppers, mushrooms, cooked spinach.

Vitamin D
From direct sunlight on the skin; also milk and dairy produce, egg yolk, fish liver oils, salmon, sardines, tuna fish. Vitamin D can be toxic if taken in excess.

Vitamin E
Whole-grain cereals, green leafy vegetables, wheat germ, vegetable oils, dried beans, asparagus.

Vitamin K
Cereals, potatoes, greens, cabbage, cauliflower, peas.

WHERE TO GET YOUR MINERALS

Calcium
Dairy produce, hard tap water, dark green leafy vegetables, Brussels sprouts, watercress, carrots, almonds, canned fish retaining bones.

Copper
Offal, nuts, dried beans and peas, shellfish.

Fluorine
Water with fluoride added, fish, most meats.

Potassium
Bananas, tomatoes, dark green leafy vegetables, bran, fish, poultry, meat.

Iron
Leafy green vegetables, liver, kidneys, dried beans, whole-grain cereals.

Magnesium
Leafy green vegetables, whole grains, nuts, soybeans.

Selenium
Whole grains, egg yolk, garlic, seafood.

Zinc
Whole grains, fish, poultry, dried beans and peas, bran, liver, eggs.

As soon as food is cooked, the vitamin and mineral content usually drops rapidly. Therefore food should be eaten fresh and raw whenever possible or lightly steamed.

DRUGS

Drugs in the right hands can be life-savers; in the wrong hands they can be killers.

We all take drugs for different reasons – to relieve pain and nausea, to help us sleep, to wake us up, to combat depression – the list goes on and on. When prescribed under medical supervision, they can be kept under control. It's when we begin taking them 'off the cuff' that problems can arise; or when we get hooked on substances that are only doing us harm.

NICOTINE

Lots of us are addicted without realizing it. Take, for example, nicotine. Smokers crave a cigarette. They're usually educated enough to know it can cause lung cancer, heart disease, etc.; they know all the facts and figures. They are probably aware that their breath is bad and their clothes impregnated with cigarette smoke and that they smell like an ashtray; but still they light up. The body becomes used to the craving for nicotine and the addiction is hard to break.

Some people are 'social smokers' – just the odd cigarette here and there – but the effect is the same: wheezing, coughing and generally being quite unfit. Smokers, with their clogged-up lungs, tend to be less energetic than non-smokers. A large inhaled breath almost knocks their socks off. They wheeze if they have to run to catch a bus and are usually the ones that miss it. If this sounds like you, don't you think you could do better than dig a premature grave for yourself? If you start exercising, this might help you to kick the habit. The two – exercising and smoking – just don't go together!

Approximately 90 per cent of deaths from lung cancer and bronchitis and at least 20 per cent of deaths from heart disease are caused by smoking. About a third of deaths caused by smoking occur in people aged under 65. And what is the point of having a firm body and a wrinkled face? Research recently carried out by ASH (Action on Smoking and Health; for address see front of book) confirms that the skin on smokers ages far quicker than that on non-smokers. It has also been found that there is hardly any difference between the skin of a 40-year-old smoker and the skin of a 70-year-old non-smoker. This applies to both men and women. The blood becomes thicker because its ability to carry oxygen is reduced.

The amount of money spent on packets of cigarettes obviously mounts up over the year. (If it's any consolation, the real price of a packet of cigarettes is virtually the same as it was in 1950, it's just the added taxation which has made the price rocket!) Therefore, if you don't feel like lining the pockets of the Chancellor of the Exchequer, isn't this a good enough reason to try to give up and line your own pockets instead?

Smoking in public is being increasingly restricted. As from January

1990, American airlines have banned smoking on all short/domestic flights, though not on all longer flights over six hours. A lot of restaurants now have a non-smoking section, and some have even banned it altogether. As a non-smoker, I applaud this action and look forward to the day when more restaurants adopt a 'no smoking' policy. There is nothing worse than enjoying a beautifully prepared meal in a restaurant and having people on the next table light up and blow smoke all over you. Personally, I have no hesitation in asking them to put their cigarettes out, but I know many people who would never dream of doing this and suffer in silence, vowing never to return to the restaurant in question. And the majority of cinemas and theatres now forbid smoking. Socially, smoking has become quite unacceptable. Don't get left behind in the excluded, unhealthy, smelly minority!

CAFFEINE
How much do you take? Perhaps you vary your drinks, from tea, to coffee, to cola, to cocoa. Caffeine is present in all these. If you're a heavy smoker and drink gallons of any of the above, your body doesn't know what is happening – one drug (nicotine) calms the system, the other (caffeine) hypes it up. If you have any history of heart problems in the family, you should beware particularly of this combination.

Try to reduce the amount of caffeine-containing drinks you take in, or you will get used to the 'high' and constantly crave more. As I explained earlier in the book, too much coffee and tea puts extra strain on the heart and kidneys and can make you feel very tense and edgy. Try instead to drink herbal teas – and, of course, don't forget the hot water with a slice of lemon – not as cranky as it sounds and very refreshing!

ALCOHOL
This can function both as a stimulant and as a relaxant. You may notice that after one or two drinks you become more relaxed, lose your inhibitions and feel 'raring to go'. After a few more, your speech becomes slurred and your vision hazy; after a few more still you could quite happily fall asleep, or perhaps go beyond this and hug the loo all night long. If you get this far, you usually wake up in the early hours feeling dehydrated and sweaty and unable to go to sleep again. This is because alcohol alters the pulse rate and blood pressure. The blood vessels open up more; hence the small red thread veins which appear on the face and sometimes the bright pink rash around the neck and chest – unattractive to say the least especially when your face becomes comparable to a blushing gargoyle!

If you do go on a bender or drink more than your usual tipple, try to drink at least two pints of water before going to sleep. This will prevent dehydration and will help the kidneys flush out the toxins.

Excess alcohol helps you put on weight just as fast as excess food. Beware of it!

PAINKILLERS

Apart from caffeine, nicotine and alcohol, there are a number of drugs which can be bought over the counter to relieve headaches, toothache, colds, flu, etc. and it can be too easy to pop a pill every time we get a twinge. If you improve your diet and lifestyle, you will very probably have fewer aches and pains and therefore be less tempted to resort to these drugs.

Drugs which are aspirin-based are used to kill pain; they will not cure it. Such drugs should never be used before exercise as obviously if you strain or hurt yourself while you are taking painkillers, you may not realize it and so may go on and hurt yourself even more.

ANABOLIC STEROIDS

Now we get on to the 'hard' stuff. First: anabolic steroids. These drugs are used sometimes by athletes and body-builders to improve performance and staying power. Anabolic steroids can be obtained relatively easily in the United Kingdom at gymnasiums and seem to be encouraged by a few trainers; at present there is little control on the sale of these drugs in the UK. It is to be hoped that legislation will be introduced if Menzies Campbell, the Liberal Democrat MP for North-East Fife in Scotland obtains a second reading of his Private Member's Bill on the misuse of drugs.

Anabolic steroids can have very grave side-effects with continued use. In a report in *The Times* (22 December 1989), John Goodbody gave evidence of the aggression factor associated with anabolic steroids: 'The effects can include an increase in aggression, violent outbursts, dramatic swings of mood, paranoid delusions and other psychiatric problems.' Certain case studies of men who had carried out violent crimes, including murder, showed that they had been taking anabolic steroids. This made them 'go over the top', become more violent and act irrationally. 'Some men exhibit over-development of the mammary (breast) glands which may not disappear entirely after steroids are discontinued. Extra breast tissue has been removed surgically for cosmetic reasons, but scarring may be visible.' Research shows that in men, the sexual drive may increase initially but after a few weeks it often decreases to below normal. And what about women? 'Women who use steroids derived from male sex hormones run the risk of developing secondary male characteristics and passing them on to a female foetus if they are pregnant when using steroids. The growth of facial and body hair, a deepening of the voice, male pattern baldness and decreased breast size all appear to be non-reversible side effects of steroid use by women which are not countered by the supplementary use of female hormone drugs.' That ought to be enough to deter you!

HARD DRUGS

Cocaine, Crack, Ecstasy, Smack, Acid, Uppers, Downers – the list goes on and on. I could sum up this section in one word: *DON'T*. Hard drugs – and drug pushers – will ruin every aspect of your life once they get a hold on you. To quote the former Home Secretary, Leon Brittan, speaking in 1983: 'We must hit the criminals who profit from the misery of drug addiction – and hit them hard. Drug abuse is a disease from which no country and no section of modern society seems immune. It brings ruthless, hardened criminals and weak, self-indulgent users together in a combination which is potentially lethal for good order and civilized values. Stamping it out will be slow and painful. The rewards are great if we succeed – and the price of ultimate failure unthinkable.'

Some of the nicest people take hard drugs and become so hooked that they can't let go. They go from one extreme of mood to another, from being quite calm to completely neurotic and totally dependent upon their 'fix'. They can also become paranoid about their health, going from bouts of vigorous exercise to abstaining to bingeing and boozing. They then become depressed, have a 'fix' to bring them out of their depression and push themselves even harder in the attempt to get back to their better previous physical state.

Users usually will look you in the eye, deny they use drugs and go along with the view that they're evil. If they are found out, they will always say they have the drug totally under control: but it never is. Continually trying to claw their way out of their quicksand pit, they find themselves being sucked down to the next fix. Their evaluation of life becomes confused and strained. They can become volatile and bad-tempered without realizing it. Their values of life go haywire.

A lot of 'high-flyers' hit the hard drugs and then find they can't get off them, with disastrous consequences. They may be very hard-working and extremely intelligent, but get trapped nevertheless in never-ending vicious circles, earning more money to buy more drugs, increasingly at the expense of everything else in their life. Eventually, they either have to seek professional medical advice; or they die – a horrific thought but a reality we should be aware of. Hard drugs are not limited to the 'down and outs'; they are supplied to the weak-willed and the big-hearted who eventually become pale shadows of their former selves purely because they can't cope without their fix: a little strip of powder becomes their lifeline and eventually sucks their life away.

Drug pushers are the lowest of the low; they get rich because they take a few risks but are rarely caught. The ones that are caught are those in the trap, the ones who take one sniff or snort or jab or whatever and find they need more and more and sell to buy. Drug pushers take lives (rarely their own) and destroy them without a backward glance, moving on to the next gullible 'pin-cushion'.

Apart from the addiction aspect of drug taking, of course, there is also the added danger of contracting the HIV virus through using other people's needles and also through generally being more careless and more relaxed when having your 'fix'!